The Best-Kept Secret in Health Care

D1472368

The Best-Kept
Secret
in
Health Care

No Drugs or Surgeries Required

Dr. Ray Drury

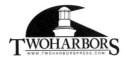

Two Harbors Press
322 First Avenue N, 5th floor
Minneapolis, MN 55401
612.455.2293
www.TwoHarborsPress.com

ISBN-13: 978-1-62652-348-7

Distributed by Itasca Books

Printed in the United States of America

Contents

Acknowledgments

To list everyone I would like to thank for their contribution to this book would be a book in itself. So, to all the people who have helped me to become the person I am and make my life as incredible as it is—thank you!

To my dad, Cliff Drury, thank you for redirecting my path to the most rewarding profession on earth. I thank my mom, Pat Delgado, for always reminding me that I can do anything I set my mind to and for helping me turn my passion into this book. To my two baby girls, Gabriella and Sophia, thank you for always reminding me what is really important in life, and to my best friend and the love of my life; Sonja, thank you for being a loving, supportive, and incredibly patient wife. I love you all.

Introduction

Patients often come to us after they've tried everything else. They've been referred, tested, diagnosed, medicated, and sometimes operated on, and they're still sick. Some have been told they'll just have to live with their pain or put up with their condition, that nothing more can be done. When these same patients are helped, sometimes immediately, by what we do, they look at us and ask two things: (1) Is it really that simple, and (2) Why doesn't everybody know about this?

Those questions get answered more fully in this book, but I will tell you now what I tell my patients; "Yes, it is that simple, and more people don't know about it because the few doctors who practice this, the ones best able to spread the word, are busy seeing patients and managing their clinics." It has not been easy for me to squirrel away the time to work on this book, but I consider it my mission in life to let sick and hurting people everywhere know there is hope for them, and it may even be down the street or across town from where they live. People suffering from a variety of conditions come to me for care from all over the world, while sick and hurting people in my own city drive by our office every day because they don't know we exist.

The form of health care about which I write has been around for over 100 years and continues to produce amazing results. My grandmother used to say, "The proof is in the pudding." It either works or it doesn't. This works, which is why it continues to grow.

The purpose of this book is to provide evidence from the clinical experiences of doctors in my profession, from patients themselves, and from carefully conducted scientific studies that proves this is, as the kids say, "for real."

Our patients have always been our best advocates, which is why our offices are mostly referral-based. When people find something that helps them heal, they want their friends and family to know about it. That's why they have voluntarily come forward to tell their stories. When someone has healed from the same health challenge you deal with every day, it gives you hope that you, too, can get well.

For example, if you're bothered by migraines, read Cynthia's story at the end of Chapter Nine. Before coming to us for care, her headaches were so severe she had to quit her job and lie quietly in a darkened room. Does your health condition limit your life because you can't trust what your body will do in public? Beverly's seizures and Patty's irritable bowel syndrome used to limit them, too, but no more. Maybe you're in so much pain that depression has set in and you sometimes wonder if it's worth pushing through the days. Read James's story at the end of the first chapter. He'd actually set a day and time to take his own life, but thanks to what you're about to learn, today James is alive and well, fully engaged in life.

All of the stories you're about to read are the true stories of real patients, told in their own words about the healing they experienced, and I know for some readers, those stories will mean more than the history, the philosophy, and the scientific studies that make up the majority of this book. Most people just want to know if what we do can help *them* like it helped their brother, sister, neighbor, or co-worker. People just want to feel good so they can enjoy their life.

I believe that if you're reading this book, there's something in it for you, or a friend, or a family member—someone you'd like to see free of a debilitating condition or pain. I wouldn't be writing this if I didn't believe with every fiber of my being that we can help you, or them, without drugs or surgery, just like I've seen thousands helped and healed over the last 20 years. I am both humbled and honored that I got to facilitate their journey to wellness, and it is my sincere hope that what you are about to read results in greater health for you and your loved ones, as well.

"The health of the people is really the foundation upon which all their happiness and all the powers as a state depend."

Benjamin Disraeli

You'd have to be living under a rock not to know that we are in the midst of a health care crisis in this country. The United States, arguably the richest nation on earth, was ranked 37th in health care systems in the World Health Organization's most current ranking.[1] One would think that the United States with its wealth and resources would have the healthiest citizens on the planet, but the truth is, we're a very sick nation. Instead of solving the problem, we seem to just keep throwing money at it.

The United States spends more on health care than any of the 12 top industrialized countries, nearly $8000 per person in 2009. Norway and Switzerland were a distant second and third, respectively, spending a little more than $5000 per person on health care. A study conducted by the Commonwealth Fund concluded that despite high costs, quality in the U.S. health care system is variable and not notably superior to the far less expensive systems in other countries.[2]

Most Americans feel they are paying more and getting less when it comes to health care, and they are. If grocery prices had gone up at the same rate as health care costs over the past 60 years, we would be paying $14.83 for a roll of toilet paper, $45.64 for a dozen eggs, and $61.66 for a dozen oranges.

Although this book is not about the health care crisis in America, it is important that we realize, individually and collectively, that what we are doing is not working. We will only get healthier as a nation when each of us starts taking responsibility for our own health. That's what this book will help you do. We cannot wait for Washington to make decisions or enact laws that will result in our enjoying better health. It's beyond the scope of what any government can do, and even if that weren't the case, we'd probably all be dead before it happened.

Today's health care treatments fall into one of four categories: surgical (surgery), pharmaceutical (medications/herbal remedies), psychological (counseling), and biomechanical (therapeutic body manipulations).[3] Each health care profession has its domain of expertise, and in order to maximize health care in America, each must be permitted to contribute where it can offer the optimum benefit to patients.

You see, we may not have the best health care system in the world, but we do have the best *crisis care* system. If you require emergency medical treatment, the United States is where you want to be.

The problem is that most of our health care needs are not emergencies. Your headache may feel like an emergency to you, but it's really not. You may even go to the *emergency* room for your headache, and you'll likely leave with a prescription that may stop the throbbing pain. But—and this is what most people don't understand— the medicine didn't "cure" the headache. The headache just appears to have gone away because the medication blocked or deadened the nerve impulses that were causing the headache. People don't get headaches because they have a Tylenol deficiency.

Nevertheless, most people have been conditioned to take a pill when they feel discomfort. We usually start with over-the-counter medications, excessive use of which has been proven harmful. If the symptoms still don't go away, we go to our primary care physician, who usually writes us a prescription. If the symptoms go away, we're usually happy until . . . they come back. Then we repeat the cycle. Most people stay in this loop of constantly treating symptoms. However, it is unreasonable to expect something *unnatural* from the outside to make things natural on the inside.

Most over-the-counter and prescribed drugs merely mask symptoms or control health problems by altering the way organs or systems work. Drugs almost never deal with the reasons why health problems exist, and they frequently create new health problems as side effects.

This so-called health care treatment results in statistics like the following: The United States, with 5% of the world's population, consumes 80% of the world's supply of painkillers, more than 110 tons of pure, addictive opiates every year. That's enough drugs to give every single American 64 Percocets or Vicodin. Pain pill prescriptions have risen 600% in the last 10 years and are responsible for more deaths each year than from heroin and cocaine combined.[4]

More than 700,000 people visit U.S. emergency rooms each year as a result of adverse drug reactions. According to the Food and Drug Administration, such reactions from drugs that are *properly prescribed and properly administered* cause about 106,000 deaths per year, making prescription drugs the fourth leading cause of death in this country.[5]

We find it upsetting that an estimated 10,000-20,000 Americans die each year from illegal drug use,[6] as we should, but when eight to nine *times* that number die from drugs that are legal we—just keep getting our prescriptions refilled? We can't blame this huge social problem on a drug cartel. Its cause is within the individuals who believe a drug will cure their physical, mental, emotional, or spiritual problems and within the institutions that have taught those individuals to believe this lie.

"We have marketed our way into this health crisis."

Frank Shorter
1972 Gold-Medal Olympian

The number of prescriptions taken by Americans increased 72% from 1997-2007 while the population during that decade grew only 11%.[7] In 2011, Americans spent $320 billion dollars on prescription drugs.[8] An estimated 65% of the country takes prescription drugs, and drugs for children have been the pharmaceutical industry's fastest-growing business. The average 18-year-old has seen over 20,000 hours of drug commercials.[9] Now *that* disturbs me. That should disturb us all.

Colleagues have told me that they have had patients suffering from migraines and patients suffering from hemorrhoids taking the same pill, usually one that is popular at the time with lots of ads on television. I've had patients who were pharmaceutical reps tell me they wouldn't take the stuff they sell.

You don't have to be an accountant to realize that the business model for medicine as it is currently practiced would suffer if patients started getting well and stopped taking some of their medications. Keeping folks on prescription drugs means the doctors don't have to go looking for new patients, and the pharmaceutical companies keep making money. Nothing wrong with making money, but the company that makes the purple pill—that's all it was called in the TV ads—made 6.3 billion dollars on that purple pill in 2010.[10] By the way, Nexium, the purple pill, treats heartburn. That's a lot of burning hearts. The pharmaceutical business is an extremely profitable one. If the purpose of all medical treatment was to get you well, their business would diminish instead of grow, and it is growing exponentially.

That prescription drugs are a huge part of America's "health care" system today is undeniable. A study done by AARP showed that Americans over age 45 take an average of four prescription drugs each day. However, what we should be asking ourselves is, "Are all these drugs making us a healthier nation?"

When medications fail to bring relief, patients are usually referred to specialists, who may recommend a surgical solution. Surgery is sometimes necessary, especially for those crisis care situations. However, reports about unnecessary surgery continue to surface. Gary Null, PhD, in his book *Death by Medicine,* reports there are 8.9 million documented unnecessary surgeries performed every year in the United States A Johns Hopkins surgeon, Marty Makary, wrote in the *Wall Street Journal* that if medical errors were a disease, they would be the sixth leading cause of death in America. These errors kill the equivalent of four jumbo jets' worth of passengers *every* week, and Dr. Makary says this is likely a conservative estimate.[11] According to the 2011 Healthgrades Hospital Quality in America Study, the incidence rate of medical harm occurring in the United States is estimated to be over 40,000 harmful and/or lethal errors each and every day.[12]

You're especially vulnerable to medical error if you're a senior citizen. According to a 2010 study by the inspector general of the Department of Health and Human Services, roughly one in seven Medicare beneficiaries can expect to suffer serious harm to their health from an adverse event during a hospital visit, and another one in seven can expect to suffer from an event that results only in temporary harm. An adverse event is defined as a "Serious Reportable Event," better known in the health care industry as "never events," because they should never happen. They include errors like operating on the wrong body part, using a contaminated oxygen line, or administering the wrong drugs. Insurance rates suggest that UPS and FedEx lose no more than one of every 200 packages they are supposed to deliver, yet estimates suggest that one in every 20 patients receives the wrong dosage of a drug—and sometimes even the wrong drug—during a hospital stay.[13]

Such data suggest that a hospital stay can be dangerous to your health. Hospital-acquired infections are alarmingly common, affecting more than two million people in U.S. hospitals and killing an estimated 100,000 each year. As David Goldhill, Harvard-educated businessman and author of *Catastrophic Care, How American Health Care Killed My Father—And How We Can Fix It*, points out, the number of people who die from infections they caught in the hospital is more than double the annual number of people killed in car crashes, five times the number murdered each year, and more than twenty 9/11s.[14] An analysis of 40 million Medicare patients' records from 2007 through 2009 showed that one in nine patients developed hospital-acquired infections, which resulted in up to $4.5 billion in additional health care expenses annually.[15]

Our current health care system is not a "health care" system at all. It's a crisis care system—a flawed, crisis care system. It's flawed because it's based on treating symptoms instead of finding the cause of disease. It is doctor controlled. (Some would argue it is controlled by the insurance companies.) It is very expensive. And it is fear-based. I see patients every day who know they shouldn't be taking all those medications, but they're afraid to stop taking them. They've been conditioned to believe bad things will happen to them if they don't take them. It used to be that drugs were prescribed for a short period, like four to six weeks. Now it seems patients are prescribed medications that they're instructed to take for the rest of their lives!

Not only is the system flawed, the premise on which that system is based is also flawed. It says, "Things are going to go wrong with you, especially as you get older. You might as well get used to it. Not only that, you're not smart enough to make decisions for yourself when these inevitable things go wrong, so someone—doctors, specialists, hospitals—will make decisions for you."

But the other side of that picture says, "You come fundamentally perfect. You have the ability to heal or recover from almost anything and to adapt to anything you can't heal or recover from." A healthy system empowers you to make your own decisions because you're the only one who knows what's true for you, ultimately.

Most people still accept without question what their doctor tells them, forgetting that they, and no one else, live in their bodies, and it will be they, and no one else, who will have to live with the side effects of a pharmaceutical drug or the consequences of a surgery that might not deliver the desired results. Patients have a right, if not a responsibility, to partner with, not just follow without question, the medical professionals they turn to for help.

A statement in *JAMA,* the *Journal of the American Medical Association*, that the U.S. medical system is the third leading cause of death in the U.S., right after heart disease and cancer, went undisputed. In fact, subsequent studies found the number of preventable deaths due to medical intervention to be *higher*. These findings are not being published by alternative health care advocates with an ax to grind. This particular article was written by a medical doctor from Johns Hopkins School Bloomberg of Public Health.[16]

Don't get me wrong. I have great respect for the medical profession and the talent and commitment most physicians bring to their work. I am not anti-surgery, and I am not anti-drugs. I wouldn't get a root canal without anesthesia, and if anyone in my family had a true medical crisis, I would rush them to the closest ER.

But what I am opposed to is a culture of health care that cuts and medicates when there are less invasive, less expensive, and often more effective approaches to getting and staying well that we either don't know about or disregard. And yes, I do oppose the misuse and overuse of prescription drugs, which is rampant in this country, especially when I know the world's greatest drugstore is in the human body. It can produce cortisone, antihistamine, cholesterol, insulin, whatever chemical the body needs, when it needs it, where it is needed, in the amount it is needed. And I oppose unnecessary surgery. I see people in my office all the time who tell me they are no better, and some say they're actually worse, after having surgery.

Perhaps some of these statistics factor into the reasons medical doctors rarely recommend alternative forms of health care, and some even instruct their patients to avoid it. Like I tell my patients, "I'm sure the candlestick maker wasn't telling everyone to go out and buy light bulbs."

The good news is a shift is taking place in this country, a patient-led revolution. Millions are seeking alternative health care. People of all ages and socio-economic backgrounds are beginning to understand that politics and profits should not stand in the way of good health, and that traditional health care should be held to a higher standard. Americans are looking for a health care system that puts their well-being first.

Alternative health solutions and natural remedies don't get advertising spots during the Super Bowl or even an honorable mention from the big pharmaceutical companies that purport to advance the health of the nation for one simple reason: There's nothing for them to patent, nothing to sell, no profit motive.

A grassroots movement usually precedes permanent change; the millions of people seeking a more natural, less invasive system to restore health is a grassroots movement, one that is gaining steam in this country. An in-person survey of 23,000 Americans conducted by the Centers for Disease Control and Prevention and the National Institute of Health shows that the alternative health field has grown by 25% in the last decade. While Americans may complain about the high cost of health care, they're still willing to shell out roughly $34 billion a year out-of-pocket on alternative treatments that aren't covered by insurance— more than they pay for traditional care.[17] Many people are combining conventional and complementary/alternative approaches. Interestingly, another study showed that only 38.5% of patients disclosed to their primary care physician that they were under the care of an alternative health care professional.[18] Why do you think that is?

The real health care crisis isn't a lack of public health care, insurance coverage, or prescription drugs. The real health care crisis is the health care system's failure to recognize that we should focus on *preventing* disease, not on treating it, medicating it, or cutting it out. We will only get healthier as a nation when we start taking responsibility of our own health. Health-conscious people have known this for a long time, and a growing number are now getting it. For those who have, and those who will, it is my privilege and duty to share what I know in my heart, mind, and soul to be one of the **best-kept secrets in health care.**

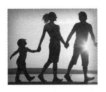

CHAPTER 1

So What Is the Best-Kept Secret in Health Care?

"All truth passes through three stages. First, it is ridiculed. Second, it is violently opposed. Third, it is accepted as being self-evident."

Arthur Schopenhauer

When people come to my office for the first time, they are often skeptical because what we do is different. It's okay with me that they're skeptical. I'm a you've-got-to-show-me kind of guy myself. I expect that many who are reading this book are also skeptical. I understand that.

The little-known health care system that has helped millions of people get their health back, the best-kept secret in health care, is *Upper Cervical Health Care*. It is a specific form of chiropractic, sometimes called *specific chiropractic,* which was developed, researched, and practiced by Dr. B. J. Palmer, son of Dr. D. D. Palmer, the founder of chiropractic. For over 100 years it has been helping people with everything from garden-variety backaches to name-brand diseases.

The nervous system is the first thing that forms in a developing fetus. The primary function of the spinal column is to protect the central nervous system, which controls all bodily functions. In addition, we depend on the spine for support and motion.

The word *specific* is crucial in understanding Upper Cervical Health Care. First, Upper Cervical deals *specifically* and *only* with the two vertebra in the neck at the top of the spine—the atlas and the axis. The atlas is named after the Greek god who holds up the world, and just like the mythological figure, your atlas holds up what controls your world—your brain. The head and the atlas pivot around the axis. The atlas and axis are found in every human being and all vertebrate animals, excluding those born with a congenital anomaly. The atlas and axis were created to support your head and protect the most vital part of your nervous system, the brain stem, while allowing for maximum movement of the head.

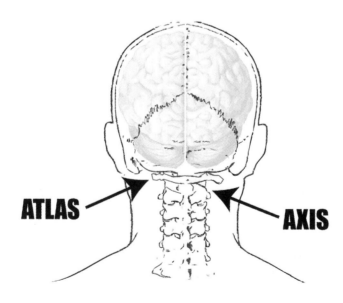

ATLAS

AXIS

The atlas and the axis differ in shape and function from the rest of the spine. The configuration of the atlas (C1) and the axis (C2) enables those two vertebrae to carry the head and to determine its movement. These articulations also protect intimate neurological and vascular structures.

The skull and its contents, which sit on top of the atlas, weigh an estimated 10 pounds. That's a lot of weight for one bone and the ligaments attached to it to support. Since some of the ligaments are lax in the upper cervical spine, the muscles play a key role in stability. Although the upper cervical area gives us the most motion—the atlas and the axis move in six different directions, allowing the head to move up or down, bend side to side, or turn left to right—this area is also the spine's weakest link.

The vertebrae of the spine below the neck have interlocking joints that limit how far the bones can move between each segment. The upper cervical spine has no bony stops. Imagine putting a bowling ball on a stack of dominoes. That's the biomechanical structure with which Upper Cervical doctors work.

"The nervous system holds the key to the body's incredible potential to heal itself."

Sir Jay Holder, MD, DC, PhD

In addition to balancing and stabilizing the head, the upper cervical spine also has a substantial influence over the body's posture and has thousands of sensors to help it perform this balancing act. These sensors are constantly monitoring the head position and making necessary changes throughout the lower spine to assure that the head remains upright.

When the spine is aligned, it is extremely strong and stable. However, due to their mobility and the fact that they're not supported or protected as well as the lower spine, the upper cervical vertebrae are less stable and more vulnerable to injury and misalignment. Plus, and this is extremely important, the part of the nervous system that connects the brain to the rest of the body, the brain stem, controls the healing process. The strength of your immune system and its capacity to fight off illness is regulated by the brain stem, and the brain stem flows through these two upper cervical bones, the atlas and the axis. Now you understand why the upper cervical spine is such a crucial area. (I find it interesting that some Eastern traditions refer to this upper cervical area as the Mouth of God.)

Neurologically, the brain stem is the most important area of the body. That's where the nerve fibers from the left hemisphere of the brain and the right hemisphere of the brain cross over. The right side of the brain takes care of the left side of the body, and the left side of the brain takes care of the right side of the body. The crossing over of these nerve fibers in the brain stem makes this a vital, vital area.

The brain controls every bodily system—body chemistry, circulation, digestion, respiration, even cognition, are all neurologically based. If you put tension or stress on the central nervous system, it's like putting a rubber band around your finger. The rubber band will interfere with the normal messages traveling though the nerves to the finger so it just doesn't function as it should. When you take stress off the nervous system, there is almost always immediate relief. You'll read about patients whose headaches, back pains, or sinus conditions went away after their first adjustment.

In other words, we know that the brain controls everything that goes on in the body, so if the brain can't communicate with some part of the body, it's going to get sick. But if the brain *can* fully communicate with all parts of the body, our body gets and stays healthy. The brain stem is like a switchboard operator constantly sending messages from the brain to the body and from the body to the brain.

It is this nerve energy that gives the body life. Some people erroneously think that blood gives the body life. Blood supplies nutrition to the body, but it is the nervous system that is the superhighway that transmits the body's life force. This life energy flows through every cell, all 75 trillion of them, and it is coordinated by the nervous system. We can live approximately three weeks without food, three days without water, three minutes without air, but not one nanosecond without nerve energy. Ask any cadaver.

Upper Cervical Care is based on the premise that when the weight of the head is shifted off the center of the neck, i.e., when there is an upper cervical misalignment, it can produce stress or pressure around the brain stem. If either the atlas or the axis gets misaligned, two things can happen. First, the bone can squeeze down on the brain stem, interfering with the healing nerve impulses that continuously travel from the brain to every cell of the body. Secondly, the area of the body serviced by the restricted brain messages will start to malfunction, possibly even shut down. That's when people get sick and disease sets in.

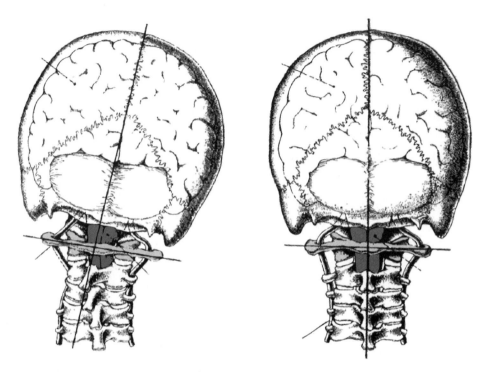

Reprinted with permission of Daniel O. Clark, DC
www.uppercervicalillustrations.com

When the atlas or axis misaligns, it can't pull itself back in. An Upper Cervical chiropractor is trained to determine if there is a misalignment in either the atlas or axis and to make a *specific* correction in this most crucial area of the spine. Since brain-to-body messages control and maintain *all* bodily functions, any interference in the free flow of these nerve impulses will impede the body's innate ability to heal.

Trillions of nerve fibers carrying messages from the brain to the body "bottleneck" through the small opening in the first and second bones in the neck, the atlas and axis, as they flow down into the spinal cord and out to every cell in the body. If the head and neck are not in proper alignment, it can cause spinal cord compression or irritation at the point where the head and neck join, which disrupts or distorts vital brain messages to any part of the body. This can cause countless health problems as well as compensatory misalignments in the upper back, lower back, and pelvis.

When there is an upper cervical misalignment and the weight of the head is moved off the center of the top of the neck, the head tilts, causing the brain to be unlevel, and the rest of the body will begin to compensate trying to level the brain. One shoulder will come down and the pelvis will tilt, bringing a leg up with it, creating a body imbalance (not a shorter leg). This chain reaction makes the spinal muscles, bones, and discs more vulnerable to injury. If your head is not on straight, the muscles from the base of the skull to the bottom of the neck, the upper thoracic area, have to tighten and shorten to hold the head up because we need the head level for equilibrium and balance. This can lead to atrophied, dried-up muscles on the anterior and hypertrophied or thickened muscles on the posterior. That is why some people frequently need to have their shoulders rubbed; those muscles are just so tight and rigid. As my colleague, Dr. Tom Forest says, "You can go to Hawaii and relax as much as you want. Those muscles will stay rigid if they have to mechanically hold your head up."

This imbalance can also result in tight, spastic muscles anywhere from the base of the head to the bottom of the feet. Over time, these compensatory changes can cause lower back pain, hip pain, knee pain—you get the idea.

That's why rather than focusing on adjusting where the pain is located, Upper Cervical doctors focus on bringing balance back to the epicenter. The atlas and the axis are the only two vertebrae in the body that do not have a means to self-correct.

"The doctor of the future will give no medicine, but will interest his patients in the care of the human frame and in the cause and prevention of disease."

Thomas A. Edison

Think of the nervous system as a superhighway of communication that flows through the atlas and axis to all parts of your body. What happens when a highway gets blocked or congested? Traffic slows down or stops altogether, right? People will be delayed in getting to their destination. In extreme situations, they may not get there at all. The same thing happens in your body. When there is interference in the normal flow of nerve impulses from the brain to the rest of the body, you get sick. If the brain can communicate with all parts of the body, you stay well.

Another analogy often used by Upper Cervical doctors is that of the water hose. Imagine that the hose is connected to its source; the water is turned on, and the water flows freely. Then you step on the hose, what happens? The water stops flowing freely; maybe now it's just trickling out. If you step off the hose, the water starts flowing again, waters the grass, and the grass grows. It's too simple for some people. They think there has to be more to it than that. We've got to spray something on the grass. We've got to put some chemicals in the soil to make the grass grow.

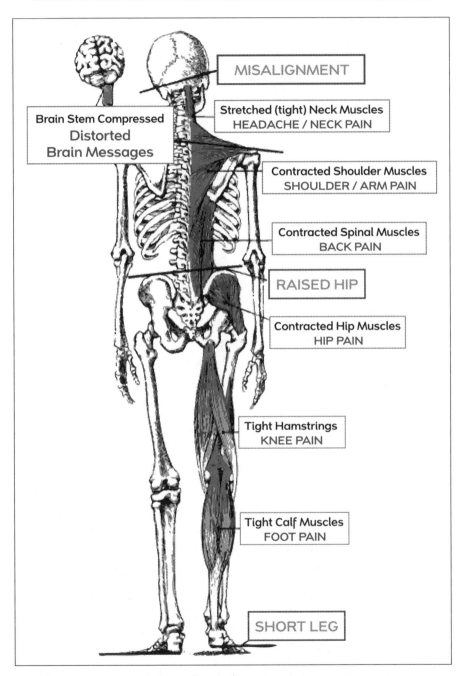

MISALIGNMENT

Brain Stem Compressed
Distorted
Brain Messages

Stretched (tight) Neck Muscles
HEADACHE / NECK PAIN

Contracted Shoulder Muscles
SHOULDER / ARM PAIN

Contracted Spinal Muscles
BACK PAIN

RAISED HIP

Contracted Hip Muscles
HIP PAIN

Tight Hamstrings
KNEE PAIN

Tight Calf Muscles
FOOT PAIN

SHORT LEG

Reprinted with permission of Daniel O. Clark, DC
www.uppercervicalillustrations.com

We have to intervene in some way. But the wonderful thing about the body is that it is intelligent within itself; it is a self-healing organism. If there's no interference, it will function as intended.

Upper Cervical doctors find the interference, correct it, and expect health. It *is* that simple.

* * *

James Tomasi, Upper Cervical Patient
Suffered from TN, trigeminal neuralgia
*Author of **What Time Tuesday?**, a book about his experience with Upper Cervical Care*

In the summer of 1986, I started having excruciating facial pain, pain that came and went without warning. It led me to withdraw to a darkened bedroom and lasted for 12 years, and for 12 years, I sought help from medical doctors, an oral surgeon, neurologists, general chiropractors, herbal remedies, acupuncture, and spiritual healers. What I got was a label for my affliction, trigeminal neuralgia, or TN, as it is referred to, and prescription painkillers that I was warned could cause liver cancer. I was told I had an incurable nerve disease for which there was no known cause.

There was no external sign to indicate where the pain was coming from, and several doctors suggested it was all in my head. One doctor used to ask me about my "phantom pain." Others made me feel I was a drug addict, just coming to them for a "fix" of prescription pain pills.

The pain was beyond description. Have you ever had a nerve exposed in a tooth? Then, imagine putting a piece of ice on that exposed nerve and not being able to spit the ice out. I just had to endure the piercing spikes that attacked my face like an electric drill. A normal day became one episode after another of pain spiking from my lower jaw to my cheekbone to the back of my head. Sometimes I was afraid to eat or brush my teeth. The pain was almost unbearable; sometimes I would scream into a pillow.

My wife, Rhonda, continued to research TN and talked to others in chat rooms online who suffered from this awful condition. We learned there were two surgeries performed for TN. One coated the nerve; another cut the nerve, which resulted in dysfunctional facial muscles. The surgeries each cost $40,000, and those who'd had them shared their disappointment that they had not delivered the relief they sought.

TN is known as the suicide disease, and after 12 years of unbelievable pain, and at this time, little hope of getting better, I decided I wasn't going to continue to live like this. So I put a small pistol in the nightstand by my side of the bed and set the time I would do it: the following Tuesday at 5:00 p.m. when Rhonda would leave the house to take our son to soccer practice. The next morning, before she went to the grocery, my wife told me not to do anything stupid while she was gone. She knew I was desperate.

On the way to the grocery, Rhonda tuned into a Tulsa radio station and heard, "Do you have pain you just can't bear? Have you been told, 'You'll just have to learn to live with it?'" The woman on the radio related how she had suffered from a debilitating pain for over 18 months and found relief in a little-known scientific technique that was so complex there were fewer than 1000 doctors in the world [who could do it]. Rhonda sat in the car outside the grocery, waiting for a name and phone number.

She rushed home to tell me about this new possibility. I was much less enthusiastic than she was, especially when I learned she had made me an appointment with a chiropractor.

"This is different," Rhonda explained. "She does an upper cervical technique, and she said TN patients had responded well to it."

"When's the appointment?" I sighed.

"Tuesday," Rhonda replied.

"What time Tuesday?"

"Ten o'clock."

I'll do this one last thing to make her happy, I thought.

The doctor took X-rays, and mindful of how painful it was for me to move my head, she treated me with compassion, which I appreciated. She took us back to look at the X-rays, and I could see that my head truly was off to the side and a little forward. She told me she was going to work on these two little bones, the atlas and the axis, that sit right below the skull. "They're not really attached to your backbone," she explained, "they just float there and that's what your head rests on."

She then told me she was going to "put my head on straight" and gave me my first upper cervical adjustment. She explained that since the disease had been years in the making, it would take some time to heal. She said she'd like to see me again on Thursday.

The pain was as excruciating as ever, and I thought to myself we'd just wasted our time and money. However, a few hours later, I woke up in my bedroom without pain. I yelled for Rhonda. The pain came back, but the reprieve reminded me what life without pain was like, and I decided to let 5:00 come and go. Instead, I went back to the Upper Cervical doctor on Thursday. Within 11 days, after three adjustments, the pain was gone, and it has not returned.

I had no idea how the little movement the doctor made worked, but I couldn't argue with the results. Now I think of Upper Cervical doctors as flipping a switch. All of us have a switch, an atlas, but for many of us, it is turned off. The Upper Cervical doctor flips that switch and this breath of life that's in our body begins to talk back and forth to all the cells, and our body heals the way it was designed to do.

Now Rhonda and I share our story with anyone who will listen. I wrote What Time Tuesday? about my experience in hopes that it will be read by people who can be helped by Upper Cervical the way I was. I believe Upper Cervical can help anyone with any health problem.

✻ ✻ ✻

* Although patients might refer to specific conditions or diseases they had when they came under Upper Cervical Care, Upper Cervical doctors do not claim to cure anything or to even treat particular conditions or diseases. Upper Cervical doctors are trained to find and correct a misalignment in the upper cervical spine, that when corrected, allows the nervous system to flow unimpeded from the brain to the rest of the body which, in turn, allows the body to heal itself.

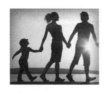

CHAPTER 2

A Brief History of Chiropractic

"First the sneer, then the cheer,
The lash, then the laurel,
The curse, then the caress,
The trial, then the triumph,
The cross, then the crown."

B. J. Palmer, the Developer of Chiropractic

It is generally accepted that the profession of chiropractic started in 1895, but the roots of spinal care can be traced back to 2700 B.C. Some of the earliest healers in history understood the relationship between health and the condition of the spine. Hippocrates, the Greek physician and "Father of Medicine," published texts detailing the importance of spinal care, writing, "Get knowledge of the spine, for this is the requisite for many diseases." Herodotus, a contemporary of Hippocrates, gained fame curing diseases by correcting spinal abnormalities.

Despite the long history of spinal-related treatments, most were crude and misunderstood until Daniel David Palmer, known as D. D., made the first spinal adjustment in 1895. Palmer had been practicing magnetic healing for a number of years and had a large following. Contrary to what the name suggests, magnetic healing had nothing to do with magnets. Rather, it was a cross between massage and meridian therapies, which is based upon the concept of acupuncture and Chinese medicine, a common therapy of the time and one that is still practiced today.

D. D. was interested in more than bringing relief to patients; he wanted to find the cause of disease. How could two people who lived in the same house, drank the same water, ate the same food, and had the same parents have dramatically different constitutions, one being healthy and free of disease and the other sickly, he pondered. Palmer believed there must be something other than environmental factors or bad luck that influenced an individual's health.

The first chiropractic patient didn't have back or neck pain. Harvey Lillard, a janitor in the same building where Palmer operated his practice, had been deaf for 17 years. Mr. Lillard told D. D. how he had been in a stooped position when he felt something give way in his neck, and he immediately became deaf. Palmer noticed a bump on Mr. Lillard's neck. D. D. had Mr. Lillard lie down, and D. D. placed his hands together and pushed on Mr. Lillard's neck to see if he could reduce the bump. After three such adjustments, Mr. Lillard's hearing was totally restored and chiropractic was born.

"Chiropractors do not treat diseases. They adjust causes, whether acquired, spontaneous or the result of injury. "

D. D. Palmer, the Founder of Chiropractic

At first, D. D. Palmer believed he had discovered the cure for deafness. The theory behind his adjustment was simple: If the lump in Mr. Lillard's neck had caused deafness, then reducing it should restore his hearing. Word traveled fast and soon deaf people from across the country were on their way to Davenport, Iowa, to get this miraculous treatment. Although he had some success in helping those with hearing loss, Palmer soon realized that many other conditions were benefiting from the adjustments he was making to patients' spines.

At first, D. D. wanted to keep chiropractic a family secret and resisted the notion of teaching others his chiropractic techniques. But in 1898, Palmer renamed his clinic the Palmer School and Infirmary and took on his first chiropractic students. His son B. J. was one of the school's first graduates.

In 1902, D. D. moved to Oregon, leaving B. J. in Davenport with an $8,000 debt and four students, but B. J. had a business and organizational acumen that his father did not have. By 1904, the Palmer School of Chiropractic was organized, and the following year, incorporated. By 1921, the enrollment had increased from four to more than 3200 students. His Lyceum, or Homecoming, as B. J. preferred to call it, brought 5,000 chiropractors "back home" every year. Besides the growth of the school, B. J. Palmer's contributions to chiropractic included extensive research, improved methods of spinal adjustment and analysis, higher standards for chiropractic education, and an increased appreciation for chiropractic worldwide. B. J. Palmer became the most significant figure in chiropractic's first 50 years, but then, as now, chiropractic had its dissenters, and B. J. battled for chiropractic on many legal and legislative fronts. He was both idolized and criticized.

One thing is certain: B. J. Palmer was a pioneer. He owned and operated the first radio station west of the Mississippi, the second radio station in the nation, and had over a million listeners a day.[19] (Ronald Reagan's first job was working at Dr. Palmer's radio station, and President Reagan was a lifelong advocate of chiropractic.)

Dr. B. J. Palmer was a meticulous researcher who worked tirelessly to uncover the scientific basis of chiropractic. He spent thousands of hours in his osteological (bone) laboratory, which grew to have over 25,000 specimens and was acknowledged by the Council on Medical Education to be the best collection of human spines in existence. Anatomy professors in several state medical colleges studied them to prepare for their own classes.

In 1908, B. J. Palmer published the first volume of what would become a series of 39 textbooks on the science, art, and philosophy of chiropractic. Known as the "green books," they are still used in chiropractic colleges today. In 1910, he introduced the new X-ray imaging technology or, as he called it, "spinography," into the Palmer curriculum. This greatly improved the science and accuracy of chiropractic care. Another major breakthrough came with the development of the neurocalometer (NCM) in 1923. The NCM replaced the old method of palpation, or feeling the spine to determine if or where a subluxation (misalignment) exists.

B. J. built upon what his father D. D. had been doing, which was basically pushing up and down on each side of the spine, popping any of the high spots. The results were some people got better, some didn't. B. J. also thought there were too many variables and inconsistencies among practicing doctors, so in 1935, he started doing research to develop and refine chiropractic techniques to get consistent, repeatable (i.e., scientific) results.

B. J.'s laboratory, the B. J. Palmer Research Clinic, was considered state-of-the-art. B. J. was a pioneer in imaging technology and the first person in the world to X-ray the spine. In 1935, it was estimated that the equipment in his research center was worth more than $1,000,000. For 16 years, from 1935 to 1951, B. J. worked on "the worst of the worst cases" that both chiropractors and medical doctors sent to him.

In the beginning, B. J. used the same method that his father had used, adjusting up and down the spine. As he began to narrow his focus, B. J. discovered he got better and better results. After 16 years of research, B. J. Palmer discovered the top two bones of the spine, the atlas and the axis, to be the cause of most of the ailments in the patients he examined and adjusted. He determined that correcting subluxations in the upper cervical spine, and in the upper cervical spine *only,* produced the most consistent, the most reliable, and the fastest results for health to return. Thus Upper Cervical Chiropractic came into being.

The B. J. Palmer Chiropractic Clinic treated over a thousand patients a day and was renowned for getting amazing results. This did not sit well with some of the local medical establishment, but it did not deter B. J., who employed medical doctors to perform a battery of 127 tests on each patient, including blood work and urinalysis, before, during, and after Upper Cervical Care to document the results and physiological changes. Over 5,000 cases of the worst conditions imaginable were recorded, validating the effectiveness of Upper Cervical Care.

"Judge me by those who know my work and I will be content."

B. J. Palmer

Patients at the Clear View Sanitarium, a psychiatric hospital in Davenport, also became part of B. J.'s research. From 1926-1961, except for an occasional violent patient who required medication, all Clear View patients received only chiropractic care from the Palmer Clinic. In 1933, doctors did only Upper Cervical adjustments per B. J. Palmer's request. The Director of Clear View, Dr. Heath Quigley, said, "The results of chiropractic care for patients were highly satisfactory across the range of nervous and mental disorders treated." The types of cases treated were 65% schizophrenia, 15% manic-depression, and 20% nervous and mental disorders.[20]

Dr. Charles Mayo, physician, surgeon, and cofounder of the famed Mayo Brothers Clinic in Rochester, Minnesota, brought his wife to the B. J. Palmer Research Center for care. The Mayos had tried every medical intervention, but all treatment had failed. Mrs. Mayo received Upper

Cervical Care for several months and went home well. A skeptical Dr. Mayo stated it was impossible for his wife to get well with what Palmer did, yet he also admitted that she was, in fact, well. After this incident, the Mayo Clinic routinely referred patients to the Palmer Research Center for care.[21]

B. J. and his wife Mabel, also a chiropractor and known as the First Lady of Chiropractic, had one child, David Daniel, known affectionately as "Doctor Dave," who lived in the shadow of his famous father for the first 55 years of his life. David Palmer graduated from the University of Pennsylvania's Wharton School of Finance in 1929 and earned his Doctor of Chiropractic degree from the Palmer School of Chiropractic in 1938. B. J. opposed his son's decision to pursue a degree in finance, but it proved advantageous, as much of David Palmer's time was spent salvaging the family's enterprises, which had suffered a significant blow in the stock market crash and the Great Depression that followed.

By the time B. J. Palmer died in 1961, he was known all over the world, had been to the White House with four different presidents, and had secured a place for chiropractic among the health sciences. David Palmer became president of the Palmer School of Chiropractic upon his father's death, transforming the corporate culture of the school into that of a nonprofit college; hence it became the Palmer College of Chiropractic. David Palmer also reinstated the full-spine model of chiropractic at Palmer College. In 1970, Dr. David Palmer, with other chiropractic college leaders, helped form the Association of Chiropractic Colleges.

D. D. Palmer was known as the Founder of Chiropractic, his son B. J. was known as the Developer of Chiropractic, and B. J.'s son David has been called the Educator of Chiropractic.

The growth of and movement toward Upper Cervical Care that B. J. so passionately promoted seemed to stall after his death, and one might speculate why this happened. For one thing, B. J.'s assertion that chiropractors needed to adjust *only* the upper cervical area was not only controversial, it was rejected by many chiropractors and even angered some. Most chiropractors were happy with the results they were getting with the full-spine adjustments that B. J. himself had taught them. Why would they want to explain to their patients, with whom they were getting these good results, that they were suddenly changing their methodology? Secondly, to convert a full-spine practice to an Upper Cervical practice would require not only additional training but the purchase of expensive equipment to make what B. J. called a "specific, scientific spinal analysis." Many chiropractors could not see the value of making that kind of investment, and those just graduating could seldom afford to.

Add to the equation the general climate for chiropractic at the time. Chiropractic colleges were beginning to seek accreditation, a legislative process, while they were also being publically scorned and ridiculed by the medical profession. Why rock the boat at a time when chiropractors needed to stand together in unity for the good of the profession? Although a decision not to promote Upper Cervical doesn't change the efficacy of Upper Cervical chiropractic, it might explain why less than 2%

of today's practicing chiropractors specialize in Upper Cervical Care.[22]

Be that as it may, Upper Cervical is still alive and well, and although its practitioners are small in number, their passion for and belief in Upper Cervical is akin to the passion and belief B. J. Palmer had for it. Exciting research that you'll read about in subsequent chapters has been published in the last 20 to 30 years, further validating the efficacy of Upper Cervical Care. Upper Cervical Health Care will not go away for one simple reason: Too many people continue to get well under Upper Cervical Care, regardless of their condition.

Lu—mother of Kevin, Upper Cervical Patient
Kevin had been diagnosed with Ménière's disease

In 1988, when Kevin was in the 5th grade, he was diagnosed with Ménière's disease. It took us a year and several doctors to get a diagnosis. Kevin was having one to two attacks every day; it was horrendous. He'd start getting dizzy, and no matter where he was, he'd just fall. He'd fall into tables, desks, whatever was around when he had an attack. Sometimes he would get nauseous, and the projectile vomiting would start. There were many days when he couldn't even get out of bed.

Our pediatrician sent us to an ear, nose, and throat doctor who sent us to an audiologist; we went from one specialist to another. Four years later, I finally said,

"Look, just send me to the best of the best," so they sent me to a doctor at Vanderbilt University who was world-renowned for his work in Ménière's disease. That doctor did the same tests and told me everything I already knew. He said the only solution was to destroy the balance nerve, which would mean Kevin would have to learn to walk again, and he could never play sports. Kevin, 13 at the time, said no to the surgery. I questioned myself later as to whether or not it was wise of me to let him make that decision.

Next, I was put in touch with a clinic in Boston that put Kevin on mega-doses of prednisone that he got so sick on, he ended up in the hospital. Then we went to Duke University where they did surgery on Kevin's right ear. It didn't help. The symptoms got worse.

Kevin had missed more than 90 days of school, and I had to fight to get him a homebound teacher. It's heart-breaking for parents to see their child so sick and watch them fight so hard. Many, many mornings if Kevin's shower wasn't turned off by a certain time, I would go to the door of his bathroom, get on my knees—to respect his privacy—and look under the door. Most mornings, I would see Kevin lying on the bathroom floor. He had had an attack.

It was clear that Kevin was getting worse. By now, he had tested legally deaf and had taught himself to read lips. He spent most of his time in bed in a darkened room.

Those were awful years. I remember holding Kevin once as he threw up, and when I reached over to flush the commode, it was full of blood. I was so scared. The hospital *visits increased right along with my disappointments.*

I decided to start a support group for Ménière's disease. I thought this would help Kevin, and it would help me. However, I soon learned there were no other children in our city with Ménière's, so my support group was made up of older people. Kevin had no interest in attending, so it became my thing.

A chiropractor contacted me and asked if he could come talk to our support group about Upper Cervical Health Care. I told him that I'd never been to a chiropractor; no one in my family had ever been to a chiropractor, but I had an open mind and was willing to have him come and let people decide for themselves.

That night I went home and showed Kevin the information the Upper Cervical doctor had given us, and Kevin said, "I want to go see him," so I made an appointment.

We had to drive an hour and a half to the Upper Cervical clinic and an hour and a half back. After two weeks, Kevin was sicker than ever. I was so upset. I called the doctor and said, "What are you doing to my son? You're making him worse!"

He said, "He's retracing. Be patient."

We were driving home from Kevin's third week of Upper Cervical Care when Kevin turned to me and said, "Mom, do you hear that?"

"What, honey?" I asked.

"All the cars driving by," he said.

I was so overcome that I had to pull off the road. Kevin could hear those cars!

By then, Kevin was a sophomore in high school. During his junior year, he missed about 30 days of school, and in his senior year, he missed 11 days and was on the soccer team. I have to admit, during that time I was walking on eggshells, afraid the attacks would come back because I had been told by everyone else that the Ménière's would never go away.

I tell people that Upper Cervical gave my son his life back.

Kevin loved college. He had been robbed of his childhood, but in college he was able to enjoy life. After graduation, he decided to go to chiropractic college. Now he's an Upper Cervical doctor in Anderson, South Carolina.

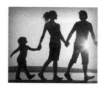

CHAPTER 3

How Does Upper Cervical Differ from General Chiropractic?

"You don't have to make anybody wrong, to be right."

My Mom

Let me start by saying I respect all my brothers and sisters who have chosen to serve the world through chiropractic. It's a worthy and honorable profession that, like other professions, has branched into distinct specialties. Today there are chiropractic nutritionists, sports chiropractors, chiropractic neurologists, pediatric chiropractors, even chiropractors for animals. They all work. I became a chiropractor because I wanted to help people, and I saw that my dad, at the time a full-spine chiropractor, was doing that.

The purpose of this book is two-fold: to let sick and hurting people know that chiropractic, in general, is a viable alternative to traditional medicine (drugs and surgery) and to let those same people know about Upper Cervical chiropractic because most people have never heard of it.

Although Upper Cervical and general or full-spine chiropractic share a common history and philosophy, there are distinct differences in the way they are practiced and in the adjustments they give patients.

In all of chiropractic, procedures are not based on the condition the patient has. They are based on whether or not the bones are misaligned which puts pressure on the nervous system and interferes with the messages the brain needs to send the body to maintain health. The primary difference between Upper Cervical and general chiropractic comes when we ask, "Which bones?" The answer is inherent in the name. Upper Cervical focuses *only* on the atlas and axis, the two upper cervical vertebrae, while general chiropractors adjust the full spine.

Upper Cervical is often called Specific Chiropractic because it focuses on this specific, upper cervical area and because it uses very specific data from X-ray analysis and other instruments designed to ensure that corrections are made that facilitate normal spinal biomechanics and neurological integrity. The X-rays in Upper Cervical offices are usually different from those found in medical or general chiropractic offices, as they allow for measurements down to a fourth of a degree to determine the exact misalignment of the top two bones in the neck and the exact repositioning that will be needed to correct it. Upper Cervical doctors believe that a very specific correction allows for maximal long-term results.

In Upper Cervical, our goal is for the correction to *hold*. Many Upper Cervical doctors prefer the word *correction* over *adjustment* and insist that the difference is more than semantics—that the two terms represent different procedures with different clinical intentions. (I will use *adjustment* and *correction* interchangeably, however.) The important distinction, for me, is that in Upper Cervical we're going after a correction or adjustment that *holds,* not something that needs to be adjusted over and over.

Upper Cervical doctors say, "Holding is healing." We very specifically correct the misalignment, then monitor that correction until it goes out again. Most visits to an Upper Cervical doctor will *not* result in an adjustment/correction; we do more monitoring than correcting. In Upper Cervical, we believe it is just as important to know when to get out of the way, i.e., when to stop adjusting and let the body heal, as it is to know when, where, and how to adjust.

Manipulating certain joint dysfunctions, as is performed by most general chiropractors has been shown to provide a valuable benefit. Most general chiropractors do full-spine manipulations, which involve moving a joint beyond its usual range of motion, but not beyond the range of motion the joint was designed to move. General chiropractors most commonly adjust the spine by using their hands to apply forceful pressure, known as high-velocity thrusts, on areas that are out of alignment or that do not have a normal range of motion. About two-thirds of visits to general chiropractors are for low back pain.[23] You can adjust a low back problem all you want, but if the weight of the head is still off-center, the minute the patient stands up, the gravitational field will take him back to the same pattern.

Upper Cervical doctors do not adjust the whole spine; we direct our focus to the upper cervical spine because if the top two vertebrae are aligned, the vertebrae below the upper cervical region can align themselves. Upper Cervical Care focuses on the specificity and precision with which an upper cervical correction is made, knowing that even a misalignment of one millimeter can adversely affect the nervous system. Upper Cervical doctors believe that a subluxation (i.e., a misalignment) has both neurological and biomechanical components, and that the spine must be studied with mathematics and geometry when considering the biomechanics of the upper cervical spine, a crucial but vulnerable area.

Again, the nervous system, made up of those brain-to-body messages, controls and maintains every single function of the body, and these messages are necessary for healing. Trillions of nerve fibers carrying these messages from the brain to the body "bottleneck" through the small opening in the first bone in the neck, the atlas, as they flow down into the spinal cord and out to every cell in the body. If the head and neck are not in proper alignment, it can cause spinal cord compression or irritation where the head and neck join and disrupt or distort vital brain messages, causing organ dysfunction and/or pain anywhere in the body—dis-ease and disorders one would not necessarily expect to have originated at the top of the neck.

"I measure success by results."

B. J. Palmer

One Upper Cervical doctor compared the difference between general chiropractic and specific chiropractic to asking someone for directions and being told to turn left at the gas station, go for about a mile, and then turn right past the house with the red roof until you come to a stop sign . . . to going to MapQuest, typing in your destination, and getting a printout with precise directions.

For example, instead of pushing a patient's hip back into alignment only to have it pull back to its old position right away, requiring another adjustment, an Upper Cervical doctor would make a correction in the atlas area to allow the muscles to reposition and restructure the spine. That's why we don't make corrections all the way down the spine. We can get the upper cervical area corrected, and it will adjust the back for us.

That's one of the unique dynamics of Upper Cervical Care. We don't chase after the pain or symptoms; we go right to the cause of the condition, the upper cervical subluxation, for which a precise correction—sometimes one millimeter, sometimes even a fraction of a millimeter—can make a huge difference. A one-millimeter misalignment of the atlas could cause asthma; it could cause acid reflux; it could cause leg pain or back pain because that one millimeter affects your nervous system, and your nervous system controls everything. That's why a specific upper cervical correction has such a powerful, healing impact.

Precise X-rays show the Upper Cervical doctor just how far the upper cervical bones are out of alignment. Without that blueprint, doctors are only guessing, and with it, they know exactly how and where to make the correction to get the bone back in place. When you have the exact angles and degrees with which to work, it doesn't take much force. That's why Upper Cervical corrections don't hurt.

Most visits to an Upper Cervical doctor will be for monitoring, not correcting. Unless objective tests tell us there's a need, we do not make a correction. Sometimes the best thing you can do for the body is give it time to heal. Holding is healing.

Many health care professionals have misunderstood the significance of treating the upper cervical spine. Some have questioned the need for specificity in the correcting of upper cervical dysfunctions. However, Upper Cervical maintains that if the cervical subluxation is causing a neurological interference, a *specific* correction is required to allow for maximal long-term results.

Most Upper Cervical doctors believe they are advancing the work of B. J. Palmer, who developed, researched, and practiced Upper Cervical chiropractic. When it comes to adjusting the spine, B. J. taught, "Less is more." In fact, B. J. taught that the upper cervical spine is the *only* place chiropractors will find a subluxation,[24] a statement that was controversial among chiropractors at the time and remains so. It is, however, the basic tenet of Upper Cervical Care.

Upper Cervical practitioners believe that when the top vertebra dislodges, the rest of the bones all the way down the spine can go out of alignment. It's called spinal compensation. When the top vertebra is put back into alignment, the muscles, through muscle memory, will literally pull the lower vertebrae back into alignment. This is called spinal decompensation. As those changes take place, the neurological pathways come back to life and the body heals itself. That is why chiropractors, all chiropractors, say that we don't cure anything; we remove the nerve interference, and the body does what it was created to do: It heals itself.

To make a precise correction to the upper cervical area requires: (1) X-rays to locate and measure the precise misalignment of the atlas and/or axis, (2) The skill to make the correction, and (3) Additional instruments that measure and produce a visual for the patient and doctor to see how much the upper cervical spine corrected after the adjustment. Often the first correction holds and the body starts healing right away, in some cases instantaneously. If the patient has had the condition for many years, the healing process usually takes longer with required follow-up care to see if the correction is holding or if further corrections are needed.

"When it comes to correcting the spine, less is more."

B. J. Palmer

Dr. James Sigafoose, a former Upper Cervical doctor who travels the world speaking on behalf of chiropractic, tells a story about a colonel in the army during Word War II who had an ankle that wouldn't heal. The colonel was sent to Walter Reed Hospital, where he was scheduled for exploratory surgery. Tests led doctors there to suspect the man had pancreatic cancer. The colonel decided to go to Davenport and let B. J. Palmer examine him. Dr. Palmer saw the colonel three days in a row, but since his first correction held, B. J. only adjusted the colonel the first day. The man went back to Walter Reed, where doctors examined him and gave him a clean bill of health. The man later served in the trenches at the Battle of the Bulge. After the war, the colonel went back to B. J. for an adjustment, but he didn't need one. The correction was still holding.

I went to chiropractic college with the intention of becoming a full-spine chiropractor because, at the time, I did not know there were any other forms of chiropractic. Then, while I was still in school, Dr. Kessinger, an Upper Cervical chiropractor who had a practice near the college, gave me my first Upper Cervical adjustment. At the time, I was what I would call healthy, although I hadn't been sleeping well and was having trouble concentrating, which I chalked up to fatigue related to schoolwork. And for the last few years, I'd had a problem with my mid-back from a high school football injury that my dad used to adjust all the time. Then there were my ever-present allergies.

When I got home from my first Upper Cervical adjustment, I slept for 12 hours, and when I woke up, my back didn't hurt. I was impressed enough that I started hanging out at Dr. Kessinger's office, asking questions, watching him work with patients, and having him give me Upper Cervical corrections when needed. I was a sponge for everything I could learn about Upper Cervical, and Dr. Kessinger generously shared his knowledge and passion for Upper Cervical Care.

After a while, I noticed I wasn't bothered by allergies anymore. Everything improved. My energy level. My concentration. My retention.

I was hooked, and my plans for the future had suddenly changed. I knew I couldn't join my dad in his practice of full-spine chiropractic as intended. I had to learn as much as I could about Upper Cervical work. I wanted to help people the way Upper Cervical had helped me. It's a decision I have never regretted.

Again, I have great respect for all chiropractors. I refer patients to general chiropractors when they want a treatment or therapy that I don't offer, and general chiropractors refer patients to me when they think Upper Cervical can help them. That, in my opinion, is how it should be. I just want people to know what we do in Upper Cervical. Then they can decide for themselves if it's something they want to look into, but they can't do that if they don't know about it.

That's why I titled the book, "The Best-Kept Secret in Health Care." In its hundred-plus-year history, Upper Cervical Health Care has always got amazing results, yet few people know it exists. Of the approximately 60,000 chiropractors in the United States, roughly 1,000 of them do only Upper Cervical Care.

Why aren't there more Upper Cervical chiropractors? We can only speculate, but here are some possible reasons: It is estimated that of the 16 years B. J. Palmer dedicated himself to work at the B. J. Palmer Research Center, the last 10 were devoted to researching, practicing, and promoting Upper Cervical Care. However, after his death in 1961, his son Dave did *not* promote Upper Cervical. In fact, it is reported that he had everything related to his father's work in Upper Cervical removed from the school. Some suggest it was professional jealousy, that Dave Palmer always resented living in the shadow of his famous father. It may simply be that Doctor Dave, as he was called, did not promote Upper Cervical Care because his gifts and interests were in the educational aspects of chiropractic.

During his tenure as President of the Palmer School of Chiropractic, Dr. Dave Palmer worked with administrators from other chiropractic colleges to secure accreditation for their schools and licensure for their graduates, which was certainly a noteworthy achievement.

Whatever the reason, the fact that Upper Cervical had lost its most famous and most vociferous advocate also meant fewer Upper Cervical chiropractors would be trained and opening practices dedicated to Upper Cervical Care.

Upper Cervical work requires either post-graduate work or specialized training. Today, many doctors graduate from college with student loan debt and need to start practicing right away. Plus, the practice of Upper Cervical Care requires expensive X-ray equipment and specialized instrumentation and adjusting tables. It costs more to open an Upper Cervical office, and doctors just starting out often have limited resources. Add to that the unfortunate fact that many chiropractic colleges have a take-it-or-leave-it attitude about working with the upper cervical spine. Today, it's possible to become a licensed chiropractor and know very little about Upper Cervical Care.

Lastly, there aren't more Upper Cervical doctors for the same reason there aren't more Upper Cervical patients: lack of awareness. If more people knew about Upper Cervical Care, there would be more demand for it, thus there would be more Upper Cervical doctors. It's a matter of supply and demand.

Some general chiropractors say they do upper cervical work *in addition to* full spine adjustments, and what they mean is they move that area of the spine. However, usually they have not had specialized training in Upper Cervical Care, so they don't have the methodology or the equipment to do the analysis that an Upper Cervical doctor has to create the very specific correction of the upper cervical bone(s). That's a crucial difference. Doing full-spine adjustments along with Upper Cervical work can actually be counterproductive. I would advise against it.

Many of the Upper Cervical doctors I talk to see Upper Cervical as a specialty within the general field of chiropractic. Seeing all chiropractors as the same is like saying an optometrist, an ophthalmologist, and an optician are all the same because they all work on the eyes. They may all work on the eyes, but they each have a different focus; they do different things and use different instruments and tools to do their work.

When B. J. Palmer was opposed for practicing exclusively Upper Cervical Care, he replied, "The world is big enough to hold those who disagree." It still is.

If you ask an Upper Cervical doctor why he chose Upper Cervical, you will probably see his/her eyes light up. Each of us has our story about how we "discovered" Upper Cervical, or how it discovered us.

There are several second-generation, even a few third-generation, Upper Cervical chiropractors who will tell you that a career as an Upper Cervical doctor was an easy choice for them. They grew up healthy under Upper Cervical Care—many of them never went to a medical doctor as a kid, not even for vaccinations.

Some will tell you they chose Upper Cervical as a profession after they had their own health restored by Upper Cervical Care, sometimes when they were children, sometimes when they were an adult in a totally different career. Just like the patients who come to them now, these Upper Cervical doctors will tell you how they had tried everything and had just about given up hope of getting better, and then they *found* Upper Cervical Care. They got well and wanted to become an Upper Cervical doctor so they could help others like they had been helped.

Then there are the converts. These are the full-spine chiropractors that, sometimes after seeing the results their Upper Cervical colleagues are getting with patients, decide to change their general chiropractic office to an Upper Cervical one. My dad would be in this category. Dad was disappointed and skeptical about my choosing to open my own Upper Cervical practice. While still in college, I drove hundreds of miles to attend lectures, seminars, and workshops on Upper Cervical Care. By the time I graduated from Chiropractic College, I was also certified in Upper Cervical.

Before I opened my practice, I went on a mission trip to Russia with other Upper Cervical doctors where we adjusted thousands of men, women, and children every day for 10 days. People were lined up 20-wide and a block long, waiting to get checked. Healings that I can only describe as miraculous happened so frequently that this was a life-changing experience for me, and I came back more confident than ever that Upper Cervical Health Care was my calling.

As the years went by, my dad and I talked more about sports than we did our work; I think we silently agreed to disagree on the subject of Upper Cervical chiropractic. Then he and my stepmom came down to visit when my youngest daughter was born. I'd just bought and furnished my dream office and was giving the family the tour when Dad turned to my stepmom, who is also a chiropractor, and asked her to adjust his lower back, explaining that a sciatic pain was running down his legs, a condition that had bothered him for years. The table was too tall for her—I use tables only for diagnostic purposes like measuring leg length—so my stepmom said, "Let Ray adjust you."

Dad said, "Can you come over here and adjust my lower back?"

"I haven't done that since I was in chiropractic school," I answered. "Look, you're in my office, why don't you let me adjust you *my* way?"

So he agreed. I ran the Tytron, an instrument that tells me if nerve pressure exists, up his neck. I pointed to the computer screen and showed Dad the nerve pressure at the top of his neck. "I believe this problem in your neck is causing the problem in your back," I told him.

I took X-rays on his neck that showed an obvious misalignment of his atlas, which was putting pressure on the brain stem, throwing his head off balance. The body was compensating by pulling one leg up short, throwing his back off, pushing the disc out toward one side, and hitting the nerve going down the leg, creating the sciatic discomfort.

I explained that I was going to correct the first bone in his neck and have him lie down for 15-20 minutes, then check him again. I knew if I corrected the position of that first bone it would remove the pressure on the brain stem and balance the head. Because his body would no longer have to compensate, his leg length would normalize, sucking the disc back into the spinal column, thus removing the pressure off the sciatic nerve, allowing the back muscles to relax and the pain to go away. This doesn't always happen immediately, but it does happen.

I knew this was my one chance to actually show my dad that I knew what I was doing and that Upper Cervical worked. So I said a little prayer as I re-scanned his neck.

The line was straight, which meant all the interference had been removed and the bone was perfectly aligned. I explained to Dad that, in time, the pain should go away.

My dad looked at me (as I held my breath) and said, "My back pain and the sciatic pain down my leg are gone."

My bravado returned.

"Well, you know, Dad, that's what we do here," I said, grinning.

I knew my dad had been having trouble sleeping for some time. When he came downstairs the next morning, he said, "I've just had the best night's sleep I've had in years."

Over the next year, my dad and my stepmom both started taking courses to learn Upper Cervical. They converted both of their practices from general chiropractic, full-spine, physical therapy practices to strictly Upper Cervical Care.

About a year later, my dad picked me up at the airport to take me to a speaking engagement I had at a Florida chiropractic college. When I finished my talk, Dad surprised me by raising his hand and asking if he could say something. Dad stood up and said to the hundreds gathered, "I did full-spine, general chiropractic for 18 years. Then I learned about Upper Cervical from my son. My two practices have been exclusively Upper Cervical for only one year, and I have had more miracle cases in which people have gotten well from all kinds of crazy conditions this past year than I had those other 18 years combined."

Years later, my dad wrote about how he experienced that time in our lives: *For many years, my son and I simply didn't talk much about chiropractic to avoid problems between father and son. I was very proud that he was a chiropractor even though we practiced differently. I chose to attend the first Upper Cervical Evolution conference because my son had put together a meeting of a large group of Upper Cervical doctors to promote unity. I thought he was delusional. This profession unified? But he had a large group of chiropractors coming, and he wanted the support of his full-spine father and stepmother, and we wanted to be there for him.*

At Evolution, we met some of the most incredible human beings we'd ever seen in our profession. These Upper Cervical chiropractors were so excited about coming together and creating this unity so they could help more people through Upper Cervical Care. It was incredible. My son and I had once half-jokingly made a deal that if he could stop my sciatica, I would seriously look at Upper Cervical.

Although I'd had a very successful practice helping patients with a high percentage of their ailments for 18 years, I had always searched for the perfect adjustment. My wife and another chiropractor had been working to stop the sciatica down my right leg for over a month with no change. I had always known how important the upper cervical area was; I had my atlas and axis adjusted many times in the past, but not with the specificity with which my son adjusted. My first Upper Cervical correction relieved my sciatica in about 15 minutes.

I had also been experiencing a lot of aches and pains that were getting a little more noticeable each year. We slept in an upstairs bedroom, and every morning I experienced sore knees going down those stairs. I assumed it was the aging process. My brother, in his late sixties, had the same complaints. About three weeks after my first Upper Cervical adjustment, my knee pain was gone! And after three or so weeks of treating my brother with Upper Cervical adjustments, his knee pain was also relieved. The stiffness in my lower back went away, and my overall health improved.

An Upper Cervical adjustment, in my opinion, offers patients the best opportunity to gain and maintain their health. That's why I want every chiropractor and every patient to understand my experience with Upper Cervical Care. I love my son, but he's not the reason I converted two practices from full-spine chiropractic to Upper Cervical. I did that because Upper Cervical Care allowed my body to heal when full-spine adjustments could not.

I believe Upper Cervical chiropractors care so much and are willing to help each other because failure in their respective offices is so rare. Upper Cervical doctors have incredible confidence in their clinics. It gives you a very secure feeling to associate with them, as a doctor and as a patient.

My dad "came to Upper Cervical" because of the healing he personally experienced after just one adjustment. I wanted to include my dad's story because he didn't seek out Upper Cervical like I did. Quite the contrary, he resisted it, doubted it, even criticized it—until he experienced his own miracle healing and wanted to be able to give back what he had received.

People are looking for a natural, easy-on-the-body, easy-on-the-pocketbook way to get and stay healthy. Chiropractic offers that.

Greg Buchanan, Upper Cervical Patient

Suffered from multiple, debilitating symptoms following a sports injury

On August 31, 1997, I was playing rugby in a Golden Oldies competition in Sydney, Australia, when I fell on my head after being tackled. I was knocked out for a few minutes, taken to the hospital, asked a few questions—what day it was, who was the leader of the country—which I answered correctly, was told I was fine and sent home. My bruised cheek and bloodshot eye soon healed, but three months later, the nightmare began.

My first symptoms included a strange pulling sensation on my right shoulder, like someone was holding me back. A week later, tinnitus (ear noises) started in my left ear. Then my head would buzz when I tried to sleep; my tongue and left corner of my mouth started to burn, and my face started going numb. Before long, I had over 40 symptoms, none of which existed prior to my head injury. One doctor told me my symptoms were just part of the aging process; I was 43 years old at the time.

For 18 months, I went from doctor to doctor and never got a diagnosis. I went to general practitioners, dentists, orthopedic surgeons, neurosurgeons, otologists, neurologists, osteopaths, physiotherapists, and otolaryngologists. They did brain scans, MRIs, cervical spine scans, X-rays, blood tests, ECGs, EMGs, ultrasounds, and Doppler carotids. All came back negative. I was told, "Learn to live with it; it's in your head," or "Take these."

My weight dropped from 190 to 132. My skin turned gray. I started to bleed from the bowel, and before long, I was bedridden. I spent about $5,000 at the Mayo Clinic. After extensive testing, doctors there referred me to a physical therapist who gave me a bunch of exercises to do.

A dentist suggested I get my C1 checked by a chiropractor. I'd never been to a chiropractor before. I was skeptical because my doctors had warned me about chiropractors, an all-too-common practice, I later learned, and in most cases totally without basis.

I'm an IT engineer; problem solving is what I do, so I began researching. By this time, my dad and I were pretty sure whatever I was suffering from was a result of my falling on my head when I was tackled in that rugby game. I researched anatomy and neurology. I read medical textbooks. I studied dissections. Then I found there was a small group of doctors in the chiropractic profession who practiced a special technique known as Specific Upper Cervical. At the time, there was one Upper Cervical chiropractor in the whole of Australia, so I went to him straight away.

When I was about halfway home after my first upper cervical adjustment, I noticed the ringing in my ears just stopped. I went home and I ate something. I felt so much better. I remember dancing around the living room with my daughter. The next morning when I woke up, I felt like a 21-year-old. It was amazing.

Ironically, the very first X-ray I had with medical doctors, they commented on my left head-neck inflection as the only thing they could see out of the ordinary. However, it was only the Upper Cervical doctor who knew the significance of this and how to correct it.

After about two weeks, all my symptoms had dissipated. It was incredible. Today the only remaining symptoms I experience I am certain are due to having TMJ surgery, something I was told would help relieve symptoms when I was having difficulty eating. The surgeon, without my knowing it, ground 4mm off my right jaw, and now my jaw is permanently misaligned. If I had it to do over, I would never have consented to the surgery.

After 25 years in IT, I resigned from Microsoft and now spend much of my time promoting Upper Cervical Health Care. I believe it is an answer to many health care problems. It helps sick people get well. It helped me and hundreds of others I have referred to Upper Cervical Care who have told me their often miraculous stories. There are thousands of anecdotal records, and now medical research is supporting the efficacy of Upper Cervical Care, as well. I've created a website, www.upcspine.com, to help spread the word about Upper Cervical, what it has done for me and others, and the research that supports it. I made a documentary called "The Power of Upper

Cervical," and I'm writing a book about it. I think the medical profession has unfairly discounted chiropractic as a viable health care system.

My last word for people who are ill but have been unsuccessful in getting results, despite seeking help from countless physicians is this: If you haven't been to see a Specific Upper Cervical chiropractor, then you may be bypassing exactly the one thing that can get you better. If you are sick and just can't seem to get well, ask yourself, "Is my head on straight?" More than likely, it is not.

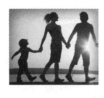

CHAPTER 4

Health and Healing Come from Within

"The body is merely a medium of expression. Innate Intelligence, is the life force. For thousands of years, professions that ministered to the sick disregarded the inside force (Innate Intelligence) and searched the heavens and earth in a vain attempt to externally find the cause of disease."

B. J. Palmer

What is health?

Let's start with the basics. To live, you need food, water, air, and something most people don't know about, which I'll, for now, call nerve energy. You can live for short periods of time without food, water, and air, but if nerve energy isn't flowing through your body constantly and continuously, you will die. Instantly.

By nerve energy, I'm referring to the energy that travels through the nervous system, a nervous system that stretches over the body's bones like a spider web. Nerve energy is the power that maintains your body. In chiropractic, we call that energy Innate Intelligence. It's an intelligence you were born with. It's the intelligence you will leave with. It's the energy that controls everything you don't consciously think about, like pupil dilation, heart rate, blood pressure, digestion, your immune system.

Innate Intelligence:

- Combines two cells, a sperm and an egg, and turns them into a unique human being with approximately 75 trillion cells.

- Tells our outer skin cells to shed and re-grow every 27 days, which means we wear about 1,000 different skins in our lifetime.

- Mends our bones when we break them. (The cast just holds them in place.)

- Knows how to operate a kidney filtering system.

- Tells the body when to secrete hormones and enzymes and in what amount.

- Takes the food we eat and converts it into chemicals the body needs.

- Tells our cells how to digest nutrients, build and repair tissues, and eliminate waste.

- Tells us to shiver when we're cold and sweat when we're hot, so that our body maintains a constant internal temperature, regardless of external conditions.

- Increases our heart rate when we walk up a flight of stairs and decreases it when we're lying on the couch.

- Activates our fight-or-flight response when we perceive danger.

- Tells babies to cry when they're hungry and to coo when all is well.

- Stops our breathing when our time on Earth comes to an end.

Innate Intelligence is our connection to the power and source that created us and knows exactly how to run, regulate, adapt, heal, and grow our bodies from conception until death. It has been called many things—the life force, source energy, the subconscious mind, and in Eastern traditions, chi. In my office, I call it God, and I've never had a single patient object to that. I see Innate Intelligence as the body's connection to the spiritual, that power which, even though we can't see or touch it, is real.

"The Innate and the educated are two separate intellects."

D. D. Palmer

Although other health care professions recognize the body's intrinsic healing abilities, having such a belief as the foundation of their practice is unique to chiropractic. The term Innate Intelligence, which B. J. Palmer always capitalized, as will I, was coined by the founder of chiropractic, D. D. Palmer. This vitalistic concept states that all life contains Innate (inborn) Intelligence and that this Intelligence is responsible for the organization, maintenance, and healing of the body. It is beyond amazing.

Let's say you eat a peanut butter and jelly sandwich that contains fats, carbohydrates, proteins, vitamins, and minerals. When you chew and swallow that peanut butter sandwich you're not thinking, *I need to push this bite down, get it into my stomach, and once there, I need to break down the carbohydrates into sugars and the proteins into amino acids. Plus, I have to break down the fats into smaller pieces, which I need to send to the small intestine. I have to secrete digestive enzymes. Then I have to get all those nutrients into the blood stream because my body has about 75 trillion cells, and each one of them needs sugar, proteins, fats, vitamins, and minerals.* How do you know which cells require what, in what amount, at any given time? Fortunately, you have this Innate Intelligence in your body that figures all that out for you, and it's a lot smarter than our individual brains.

Innate Intelligence is our spiritual life force. It's the energy that animates all living things. We wouldn't be here if we didn't have it. Upper Cervical Care is not just a philosophy. It's not just a theory. It's not just a belief system. Upper Cervical Care is also a science. So if it's a science, how do you *prove* Innate Intelligence? How do you prove God?

Well, your body is made of an estimated 75 trillion cells and at any one moment in time—and a moment is not a measurement of time but more of a slice through time—approximately 200,000 chemical reactions are going on in each cell. How many chemical reactions is your body experiencing in one moment? Seventy-five trillion cells x 200,000 chemical reactions = a number larger than I know how to write. Now, try to imagine how many chemical reactions occur in your body in 60 seconds, in an hour, a day, a week, a month, a year. We're approaching infinity, right? Which I think is pretty cool, but what's even cooler is that every single one of those chemical reactions has a specific purpose.

If all this is happening for a reason, then there has to be organization in the body, just like there's organization in nature. Seasons cycle with certainty and regularity, as does night and day and the ebb and flow of the tide. Things don't happen haphazardly or at random. If there's organization, then there has to be intelligence. Have you ever seen a house just accidentally build itself? So if we have infinite chemical reactions that are organized, we're dealing with Infinite Intelligence. The only thing that is infinitely intelligent is God.

Let's go back to the question, what is health? If we define health as a 100% expression of Innate Intelligence through the body, a 0% expression of Innate Intelligence would be death, so most of us function somewhere between 0% and 100%. A steady diet of junk food can lessen our expression of Innate Intelligence as can smoking a couple packs of cigarettes a day. Trauma experienced due to illness or accidents can interfere with the body's full expression of Innate Intelligence, as can stress.

Your body is matter, and it's not alive until Innate Intelligence passes into and flows through it. This intelligent force is the essence of life, which gives you the *innate* ability to heal, grow, and transform. It knows how to direct the body toward optimum health, provided the path—the nervous system—is unobstructed. If the neural pathway is clear, then healing messages will reach every one of the body's trillions of cells at 100% capacity, 100% of the time. However, a subluxation can significantly reduce our expression of Innate Intelligence and—obstructs the flow of this nerve energy that keeps you well without your knowing it, and it's the work of the Upper Cervical doctor to see if this subluxation is present in your body.

Remember that if you cut off the nerve supply to any part of the body, it will die. For example, if you cut off a finger and set it aside, that finger will die. Even if you somehow maintained the blood supply to the severed finger, it would still die. Blood nourishes the body, but it's the nervous system that gives it life. If you cut off the nerve supply to any part of the body, it will die, regardless of how much food—fats, carbohydrates, proteins, vitamins, or minerals—you give it. Food nourishes the body; it takes a long time for a part of your body to starve to death. It takes no time for a part of your body to die if you disconnect it from the source, from Innate Intelligence that manifests in the body as nerve energy that travels via the nervous system.

A subluxation is when one of the top two bones of the neck, the atlas or the axis, misaligns to the point that it puts pressure on the nervous system, interfering with the normal transmission of nerve impulses from the brain to the body and from the body back to the brain. This misalignment obstructs the flow of Innate Intelligence, which means those impulses will not get to the parts of the body they would have if there had been no obstruction. When the body does not get what it needs, in time, symptoms develop. That's why in Upper Cervical we say, "Symptoms are good." They signal to us that something is not working as intended so that we can address the problem at hand.

Let's use the pancreas as an example. Let's say you ate a piece of candy that sent sugar to your stomach. A message travels from your stomach to your brain through the nervous system and tells the brain that you have sugar in the body. The brain responds by sending a message down to the pancreas that says, "Hey, we've got sugar in the body; we need insulin pumped into the bloodstream to get the glucose (sugar) and take it to the parts of the body that need it now." Understand that the message goes from the brain *down* to the pancreas. If the message leaves the brain at 100% capacity, goes through the brain stem, down the nervous system, to the pancreas, and delivers the message at 100% capacity, then the pancreas functions at 100% capacity.

However, if the atlas or axis is misaligned to the point that it interferes with that message getting from the brain to the pancreas, now the pancreas gets less than 100%— who knows how much less than 100%. We do know that *anything* less than 100% will keep the pancreas from functioning normally. Let's say the pancreas is not producing the proper amount of insulin, so you go to your medical doctors and they see only the effect. They don't see that the pancreas is not performing as it should because it's not fully communicating with the brain. They see that your body is low on insulin, so they treat the *effect* by giving you insulin to take. Now, that is going to help you process the sugar in your body, but is it ever going to fix the underlying cause? No.

What if you have an upper cervical misalignment that is cutting off some of the nerve supply to the bronchial tubes, and they're not dilating like they're supposed to? You can get symptoms we have grouped and labeled as asthma. What if the upper cervical misalignment is impeding the flow of nerve energy to the colon? You might get constipated and, over time, get diagnosed with irritable bowel syndrome. Let's say the communication from your Innate Intelligence is not getting to your stomach at 100% capacity. If that happens, you might not be able to process your food properly, and you might get what we have labeled acid reflux, colitis, or heartburn.

An upper cervical misalignment could impair Innate Intelligence's communication to your heart. What does a heart attack feel like before it happens? Usually nothing, because it takes about 10 years for a heart to get diseased enough to stop beating or to bring on a heart attack. So you could have nerve interference to your heart for many years, and you wouldn't know it because it takes so long for symptoms to appear.

Interestingly, we have no nerves that come off of the brain. We do, however, have 12 cranial nerves that come off of the brain stem and go back up and innervate the head, face, and neck. Interference to these cranial nerves can affect your vision, taste, or smell. It can cause dizziness, vertigo, and hearing loss. Nerve interference can affect the trigeminal nerve, which gives a sensation of pain in the face when there's actually nothing wrong with the face.

The brain is an organ, just like the pancreas is an organ, the kidney is an organ, etc., and each organ has a function. The brain's primary function is processing thoughts, memory, emotions, and conscious awareness. When you have a thought, memory or emotion, it travels from the brain down to the brain stem. The brain stem, like a switchboard operator, sends a message to another part of the brain that interprets it. If there's an interference of the nerve energy at the level of the brain, that message doesn't get fully communicated, which can result in altered emotions, such as depression, anxiety, or panic attacks. It can affect knowledge retention, creating conditions we have labeled as attention deficit disorder (ADD), attention deficit hyperactivity disorder (ADHD), dyslexia, or dementia. A misalignment at the brain stem, where the upper cervical bones are located, can interfere with transmissions from the brain *to* the brain and cause mental, emotional, or learning problems.

That's why Upper Cervical doctors look inside your body to determine if you have a misalignment that could be interfering with the normal healing process you were born with, Innate Intelligence. If so, we can remove that interference and the normal messages will now travel through your body, healing your body and keeping your body well. This is how Upper Cervical Care is able to help sick people, regardless of their condition. It is also why Upper Cervical Care is one of the best ways to maintain health. It is a wellness approach to health care that puts nothing in the body and takes nothing out of the body. We don't treat symptoms; we locate and correct the cause of the health problem, which allows the body to heal itself.

"The power that made the body is the power that heals the body."

B. J. Palmer

The human body is both amazing and amazingly complex, with approximately 75 trillion cells serving different parts of the body, performing different but crucial functions. Yet every bodily function is conceived, organized, and instructed by this unseen intelligence, Innate Intelligence, inside each of us that operates every second of every day without our conscious awareness.

When all the cells do their job, the body is balanced and healthy. Innate Intelligence doesn't need our help to perform, since, being spiritual, it is perfect. However, Innate Intelligence works in physical matter, the body, which is not perfect. Unlike our spirit, matter is limited and subject to the forces of time, gravity, and all kinds of stress. These can interfere with the normal and natural flow of Innate Intelligence by way of the nervous system to the cells, tissues, organs, and systems of the body. When this happens, the body gets out of balance, creating pain and disease.

This happens because the nerves bring critical information and nutrients from the brain to every cell. That's their job, 24/7. Upper Cervical doctors believe, as B. J. Palmer did, that the upper cervical spine is the most crucial area of the spine since the atlas and axis are positioned right next to the brain stem through which all nerves have to flow on their way to and from the brain. We believe that the wisdom from within—Innate Intelligence—is "unlocked" most precisely by an Upper Cervical correction.

"Healing comes from above-down, inside-out" is an often-repeated phrase in chiropractic. It is based on beliefs about the human body and the natural order of the universe. This sets chiropractic apart, for many professions are not based on a set of principles. The legal profession, for example, deals with laws, not principles, because laws change with time, location, or society's preferences. During the gas crisis, many interstate speed limits were reduced to 55 MPH. Today, you can legally drive 70-75 MPH on those same roads. Medical practices change. MDs used to remove tonsils as a preventive measure. Today, tonsillectomies are rare.

Chiropractic is based on the principle that the body has the ability to heal itself, and principles don't change. They're just as true today as they were 50, 100, or 1000 years ago. They worked yesterday, they work today, and they'll work tomorrow. They work for the two-year-old toddler, the 40-year-old firefighter, and the 70-year-old grandma. You don't even have to believe in it for it to work. If I had a dollar for everyone who said they didn't believe in chiropractic whose body healed anyway under chiropractic care, I would be a very rich man.

So, Innate Intelligence not only knows how to create a human being, it also knows how to maintain one, and will do so at optimal levels unless this life force, for which the nervous system is the conduit, is obstructed. The chiropractor's work is to locate, evaluate, and remove the obstructions (subluxations) to the nervous system, so the body can do what it was created to do: Heal itself.

Doctors don't heal. Medications don't heal. Operations don't heal. Chiropractic adjustments don't heal. All *any* doctor, pill, procedure, or adjustment can do is to remove the *interference* to healing, so that the body's own Innate potential can be expressed, above-down, inside-out.

"Our inner intelligence is far superior to any we can try to substitute from the outside."

Deepak Chopra, MD

I am continually surprised and humbled as I witness what Innate Intelligence can do for people, many who have suffered for years, when an Upper Cervical correction unlocks their nervous system, allowing it to flow unimpeded to every cell of their body. That's what happened when D. D. Palmer adjusted Harvey Lillard's neck in 1895. Mr. Lillard's hearing was restored, and chiropractic was born.

At its inception, chiropractic embraced the belief that all life contains an unchanging and unchangeable Innate (inborn) Intelligence and that this force is responsible for the organization, maintenance, and healing of the body. I'm sorry to say that not all chiropractors still accept this vitalistic philosophy. Today, some chiropractors may have never even heard of it because some chiropractic colleges are no longer teaching it. They prefer to align with the medical model of treatment, training chiropractors to function similarly to physical therapists that work in medical facilities. You will find some chiropractors who now define Innate Intelligence as homeostasis, the ability or tendency of an organism or cell to maintain internal equilibrium by adjusting its physiological processes. Others see Innate Intelligence as a way of referencing the unexplainable, similar to the way we attribute certain phenomena to "Mother Nature." They think chiropractic's belief in Innate Intelligence sounds too spiritual, too metaphysical, too religious, or too "unscientific." Joseph Keating, PhD, said of Innate Intelligence, "The belief in immaterial intelligence is a matter of faith, not science,"[25] a statement that presupposes faith and science cannot coexist.

You've probably surmised from my tone that I'm not in that camp. I believe wholeheartedly in the healing power of Innate Intelligence in the human body, and in life in general, and I count on it to do its healing work in my patients every day. And as you can tell from the patients' stories you've been reading, Innate Intelligence is doing that. I'm just happy to be a facilitator in the process.

Who am I to determine what can and cannot happen? Who am I to tell patients that the Innate Intelligence within them, that created them from two cells, can heal them of some things but not others? I learned early on not to take on that role. It's not my job to play God. It's my job to know when, where, and how to move the bone. How Innate Intelligence heals people, at what rate, and in what time frame is unknown to me. I just trust, believe, and therefore know healing happens. I, and every Upper Cervical doctor I know, have witnessed too many patients getting well to doubt this.

In his book *Quantum Healing,* Deepak Chopra, MD, stated that when he researched and thought about Innate Intelligence and medical intervention, he came to three conclusions:

- One, that intelligence is present everywhere in the body.

- Two, that our own inner intelligence is far superior to any we can try to substitute from the outside.

- And three, that intelligence is more important than actual matter in the body, and without it, that matter would be undirected, formless, and chaotic.[26]

Upper Cervical doctors say, "We move the bone; God does the healing." We remove the interference, thus allowing your inborn, God-given healing potential to express itself throughout your body, helping your body to normalize and heal. We who are honored to do this work like to say, "Upper Cervical adds life to your years and years to your life."

✳ ✳ ✳

Beverly R., Upper Cervical Patient
Suffered from seizure disorder

I'd been having seizures for 13 years when I came to Upper Cervical. I would have six to eight seizures a week. They would just come out of the blue. I never knew when I would have one. In fact, I had a seizure in the office during my first Upper Cervical appointment when the doctor was X-raying my neck. I fell right out of the chair.

The Upper Cervical doctor explained how the nervous system works in the body, and everything he said made sense to me. I felt kind of faint after my first adjustment, and when I lay down, my leg went numb and my head felt weird. I just felt kind of weird all over, not hurting, just weird. When I got up and the doctor re-checked my neck, he told me he thought my upper cervical had loosened up from the position it had been kind of frozen in. I have not had a seizure since that day, not since my very first Upper Cervical adjustment. That was over six months ago.

At first, I thought that this Upper Cervical doctor would be just another doctor I went to. I'd been to too many medical doctors to count and to four different chiropractors, but none of them were Upper Cervical chiropractors. One of them did adjust my neck. He told me he did Upper Cervical, but he just pulled and twisted my neck, which hurt. I didn't go back to him. His adjustment wasn't anything like that of the Upper Cervical doctor I go to now, who has really helped me. He does nothing but Upper Cervical adjustments.

I hurt my neck in a car accident when I was 16. I think the trauma of that neck injury had something to do with the seizures I've had over the years.

When I came in today, I had an awful migraine. My Upper Cervical doctor thinks I'm retracing because I used to have migraines. But after he adjusted me, my migraine went away. As I rested after the adjustment, I could actually feel my headache roll up and out of my body. It's hard to explain. I just know I feel so much better than when I first came in. That's why I try not to miss an appointment. People say, "Why do you drive over an hour to see your chiropractor? We have plenty of chiropractors here." I tell them, "But they're not Upper Cervical."

I think a lot of people don't understand Upper Cervical because when I tell them my doctor adjusts the neck, people automatically think their head's going to be pulled and jerked or twisted around, but that's not what happens. I try to tell people, with Upper Cervical they find the exact spot to adjust and then put a little pressure on that exact spot to get the atlas and axis back in alignment. [My doctor] does this until the adjustment holds. I'm seeing my Upper Cervical doctor once every two weeks now, and the last time I came, I didn't have to get adjusted, so I'm beginning to hold my adjustments longer.

Before I came to Upper Cervical, my doctor had me taking a lot of meds, but I'm gradually getting off of them.

The last 13 years have been really hard. I just never knew when I'd have a seizure. One time I had a seizure on my porch, and someone passing by saw me lying there and called an ambulance. I've been taken to the hospital in an ambulance after I've had a seizure many times. I was always afraid to leave my house, afraid I'd get out somewhere and have a seizure. When I had a seizure I'd shake uncontrollably; sometimes I would vomit. It was embarrassing.

I haven't been able to work or to drive. If I can go a year—six more months—without having a seizure, I can get my driver's license again. I'm so looking forward to being able to go where I want to. For a long time I've been a prisoner in my own house. Now, just to be able to go to Walmart or to my mother's house on Sunday without me having to worry about whether or not I'll have a seizure, it's a treat, I tell you. To go to church and know I can stay for the whole service, that I don't have to sit there afraid that I'll have a seizure. Things that probably sound like little things to most people mean a lot to me, because for so long, I couldn't do them.

I'd just like for people who are having seizures like I did to know that Upper Cervical is a great find. When I first came here, I didn't expect Upper Cervical to be able to help me, but it did. Maybe it will help them, too.

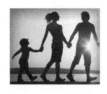

CHAPTER 5

An Art, a Science, and a Philosophy

"During human progress, every science is evolved out of its corresponding art."

Herbert Spencer

The general concept of chiropractic care is based on the universal law of cause and effect. For every effect—symptoms of mental or physical ailments—there must be a cause. Doctors of chiropractic focus their efforts on locating and correcting the cause of the patient's condition, allowing the body to heal itself naturally without the use of potentially harmful drugs or surgery.

Chiropractic, like most professions, has a vernacular that grew out of the history of the work; this vernacular is seldom used by the general public. One such word is *subluxation,* which I have already used but will now define in more detail. B. J. Palmer made a distinction between a subluxation and a misalignment. He wrote, "Subluxation, more than a misalignment, is a condition of three correlated vertebrae which have in part lost their normal relationship in juxtaposition... where it *does* produce pressure upon nerves, *does* interfere with or create resistance to the transmission of mental impulses between the brain and body, and *does* hereby become the *cause* of dis-ease in one or multiple places in the body."[27] B. J. is saying that a vertebra may be out of alignment with the vertebra above or below it and *not* be a subluxation. The misalignment must be producing pressure on the nerves and interfering with the normal flow of the nervous system to be a subluxation that causes dis-ease in the body.

Therefore, a misaligned vertebra or vertebrae is merely a compensation unless it is accompanied by neurological interference. It is believed that each individual has a range of misalignment tolerance before significant neurological interference occurs. The effect of restoring neurological integrity through the correction of a vertebral subluxation on one's health and well-being should not be underestimated.

It has been determined clinically that degeneration tends to occur around areas of biomechanically unstable joints, and the C1 (atlas) and C2 (axis) are certainly that. When the upper cervical vertebra(e) are out of alignment, which Upper Cervical doctors determine by X-ray and other equipment, a dysfunction (subluxation) can develop to which the body must continually adapt from a biomedical standpoint. This is due to the connective tissue damage that usually occurs when a force causes a trauma to the supportive structure.[28] It is generally recognized that the original cause of an upper cervical subluxation is trauma. This would result in ligament and joint damage. The sources of the trauma that cause the damage to the upper cervical area can be many and varied—everything from the trauma one experiences during the birthing process to trauma from falls, accidents, or other injuries.

This is important to understand because the art of Upper Cervical Care is in the practitioner's ability to locate, diagnose, and correct the *subluxation(s)*. Chiropractors study and practice a variety of techniques to help them do this, and the art with which they practice depends on a lot of factors: their education and experience in chiropractic in general and Upper Cervical in particular, their training and experience in the particular technique they use for correcting the subluxation, the equipment and instruments that help them make specific and accurate corrections—even their commitment to Upper Cervical and helping sick people get well influences the artistry individual doctors bring to their work.

Chiropractic is also a science, although there are those who will argue it is not. Let's explore this. Science is usually defined as the systematic pursuit of knowledge involving the recognition of a problem, the collection of data through observations and experiments, and then the testing of a hypothesis. Chiropractic meets this definition, and later in this book, you will see a sampling of the mounting scientific evidence from published research that proves Upper Cervical chiropractic works.

For me, it's as simple as this: any method or procedure can be called *scientific* when a particular set of criteria produces consistent results. Upper Cervical doctors will tell you that is what they appreciate about *specific* chiropractic, that they consistently see patients improving and healing under Upper Cervical Care, regardless of the condition or diagnosis the patients had when they came into their offices. Chiropractic is based on the *scientific fact* that the nervous system regulates every cell, tissue, organ, and system in the body.

For over a hundred years, many in the medical profession have rejected chiropractic on the basis that it is not scientific, even though some of the research studies that prove the effectiveness of chiropractic care have been done by their own medical institutions and their own medically-trained physicians.

The truth is, very little in the health care professions—or any profession, for that matter—can be proved beyond a shadow of a doubt. Dr. David Eddy, MD, PhD, while a professor of Health Policy and Management at Duke University, concluded, "Only about 15% of medical interventions are supported by solid scientific evidence... This is partly because only 1% of the articles in medical journals are scientifically sound."[29]

By most accounts, it appears that the framework for medical research is flawed. Dr. John Ioannidis, the chief of Stanford University's Prevention Research Center, states that there is less than a 50% chance that the results of any randomly chosen scientific paper will be true. According to his study, "Simulations show that for most study designs and settings, it is more likely for a research claim to be false than true."[30]

Dr. Marcia Angell, in her book *The Truth About the Drug Companies: How They Deceive Us and What to Do About It*, exposes many examples of why medical studies often cannot be trusted, stating flat out: "Trials can be rigged in a dozen ways, and it happens all the time." Dr. Angell is the former Editor-in-Chief of the *New England*

Journal of Medicine and a Senior Lecturer in Social Medicine at Harvard Medical School.[31]

"There is a vast difference between treating effects and adjusting the cause."

D. D. Palmer

Yet medical doctors' big complaint against chiropractic for years has been that chiropractic doesn't have the science to back up its claims, and *that* is just not true. (See Chapter Nine.) However, it is understandable that to the uninformed, an Upper Cervical correction appears rather "low-tech" compared to, say, an MRI scan. (One MRI machine, by the way, costs over $1,000,000.) It's also true that a chiropractor will not write you a script for the latest and greatest drug that suggests you, too, can be happily running through fields of wild flowers like the usually beautiful and usually young woman in the drug companies' ads. You know the ones I'm talking about— the ads that mumble a long list of the drug's possible side effects at lightning speed. If you really believe drugs or surgery—both important and sometimes necessary, although not to the extent they're used—can make you healthy, then you're wasting your time reading this book. Chiropractic is based on an entirely different premise, one that's unique among health care practices: If your body is getting what it needs, it *can* and *will* heal itself.

The philosophy of chiropractic is one of my favorite things to talk about because chiropractic doesn't *have* a philosophy; chiropractic *is* a philosophy. Chiropractic is more than a belief; it's a way of life. The Innate Intelligence that you just read about is the foundation for that belief system, which manifests always and in all ways.

In medicine, diseases are complicated and multiple; causes are multiple; cures are multiple. Medicine focuses on the diagnosis of symptoms. In chiropractic, we don't treat diseases or symptoms. We're not even all that concerned with what they are. Our focus is on the analysis of cause. Medicine's success is in the treatment of disease, not in restoring health.

B. J. Palmer was in great demand when he was treating patients. Then, like now, people wanted to go to the best. (That's why Dr. Mayo took his wife to Dr. B. J. Palmer.) B. J. used to get impatient with people who came to see him because they'd want to go through a litany of everything that was hurting, what the doctors had said was wrong with them, and all the things they'd done that hadn't helped. He would bluntly tell patients that he didn't need to know any of that and that they were taking valuable time away from other patients he could be helping. He explained, just like Upper Cervical doctors still explain to patients, that if he found a subluxation and corrected it, they should get better, regardless of their condition or disease. A balanced spine and nervous system are important regardless of the patient's condition.

Not one person has ever been "cured" by a doctor. A physician, any kind of physician, can only remove the obstacles to health. In chiropractic, the obstacle to health is nerve interference. Based on the premise that the body is a self-regulating and self-healing entity, Upper Cervical doctors detect and correct a subluxation in the upper cervical spine, which allows nerve impulses to now flow unimpeded from the brain, through the brain stem, down through the spinal cord, and then literally to every cell of the body. Innate Intelligence directs this flow of energy, which does for our body whatever our body needs it to do. Our body, through the power of Innate Intelligence, knows what it needs to be healthy and fully functional.

For me, this is the proper order: Chiropractic is first a philosophy, for without the healing power of Innate Intelligence, the chiropractor's work would be in vain. Secondly, it's a science. To be a viable health care practice, chiropractic must be safe and produce good results that can be duplicated and repeated. It does this, so chiropractic is a science. Finally, the art of chiropractic comes in the skill of the practitioner and in the accuracy and precision of the adjustment or correction. Upper Cervical doctors get trained in specific techniques that help them develop the art of Upper Cervical Care.

✳ ✳ ✳

Theresa R., Upper Cervical Patient
Diagnosed with multiple sclerosis

Before Upper Cervical, I had migraine headaches for 15 years. However, doctors never diagnosed them as migraines because the medicine they prescribed for me, drugs that were supposed to treat migraines, never worked. So I walked around every day with this excruciating headache. In 2009, when I temporarily lost sight in one eye, I was diagnosed with multiple sclerosis.

My neurologist explained to me there are different forms of MS. For some people, MS is crippling; he said he had one patient with MS who couldn't control his bowels; some people with MS look as if they've had a stroke. Symptoms of MS appear and often disappear as mysteriously as they came, and that's part of the fear factor—you don't know what's going to happen today. You can go to bed fine and wake up in the morning and think, "What in the world?" I never even told my family that I'd been diagnosed with MS because mothers have a tendency to worry, and people don't realize the kind of energy they're putting around you by worrying. My family still doesn't know I was diagnosed with MS.

Now, I consider the diagnosis a blessing because it made me question why I am here, to start asking questions that, up to that point, I'd never even thought about. I was just living my life, day to day.

The doctors could not give me any answers about who, what, when, or why as it related to my having multiple sclerosis, so I had to seek answers for myself. I knew MS was a disease that attacks your central nervous system, which controls everything in your body, so that's why it affects people differently. My search resulted in my finding Upper Cervical Care. I have learned that if you ask, the answer will show up.

I had my first Upper Cervical appointment in late 2009. The Upper Cervical doctor X-rayed me and gave me some information that made so much sense. My first question to him was, "Why doesn't my neurologist know this?" I'm a science-type person, and Upper Cervical made complete sense to me. It also gave me something to believe in, something to hold on to.

My headaches went away immediately after my first Upper Cervical adjustment. I remember waking up and thinking, something's different, and then I realized I didn't have a headache! Even though the relief was immediate, I continue to stay under Upper Cervical Care to stay healthy. My appointments have gone from three times a week in the beginning, to now I come every other month to be checked. I'm able to hold the adjustment really well now, and I feel good. It's wonderful.

I met another patient who had been diagnosed with MS the last time I came to see my Upper Cervical doctor, and we talked about how MS can mess with your mind. You never know what's going to happen to your body next, what symptoms you'll have, and when or if they'll go away. It's easy to start feeling sorry for yourself; you can get depressed and feel hopeless because nobody can answer your questions about MS. I mean, when doctors tell you they don't know what causes it, that there's no cure for it, and that they don't know if the medicine they're giving you is going to work or not, you have to be mentally strong; there are so many unknowns.

That method of treatment didn't work for me, but the theory behind Upper Cervical, its explanation of why my body wasn't working the way it was supposed to, made perfect sense, and for me, Upper Cervical has worked perfectly. I don't take my MS medicine anymore, and I suffered no ill side effects when I stopped taking it. I never believed it was any kind of cure that was going to help me in any way, and quite frankly, I didn't know what that crap was that they were having me shoot up in myself.

Upper Cervical, for me, has been a solution, one that didn't involve taking drugs, which, you probably figured out, I do not like taking. We have been so duped into believing that doctors are our saviors, and they are not. They have been trained to identify symptoms and label those symptoms as particular diseases, then medicate or operate.

Today, I have a completely different mind-set. That, along with Upper Cervical Care, has totally healed me. I would tell people to do their research and give Upper Cervical Care a try, especially if they are like me and don't want to give themselves a shot every day. There's an alternative that doesn't require that. It just requires an open mind. Even my neurologist said, when I told him about my success with Upper Cervical, "Whatever works for you." Now, he's an open-minded medical doctor, but I think that should be the mindset of every health care professional—whatever works for the patient.

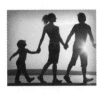

CHAPTER 6

Upper Cervical Care Embraced by Europeans

"Build it and they will come."

Field of Dreams, movie

In 2007, after 15 years as an Upper Cervical doctor, I had achieved most of the goals I had for my practice. I had three large practices with four Upper Cervical doctors working for me. I felt I had made a positive contribution to my city through Upper Cervical Care; most people would look at my work and call it successful. At the same time, I grew restless thinking of the millions of people all over the world who were sick and suffering, taking unnecessary medications with harmful side effects, and possibly scheduled for needless surgeries, who had never heard of Upper Cervical Care. I knew in my heart so many of them could be helped by Upper Cervical—if they only *knew* about it.

So I turned my clinics over to my other doctors, took a leave of absence from my practice, and with my partner, Dr. Thad Vuagniaux, created Upper Cervical Health

Centers, Inc., with the intention of linking Upper Cervical clinics across the country, then functioning like little islands. The goal: to introduce the world to the benefits of Upper Cervical Care. This career move was a giant leap of faith, as we would be trying to launch an international movement on a shoestring budget.

Coincidentally, or some might say serendipitously, within months of my leaving my practice, I started getting calls from Italy, from friends and relatives of sick people, sometimes from sick people themselves, who had heard about Upper Cervical Care and wanted to come to the states to see if I could help them. I explained that I wasn't currently seeing patients, but they were insistent. By the end of one year, I had 18 patients from Italy, some who arrived in Charlotte so sick they had to be brought to my office from their hotel by ambulance. Like B. J. Palmer, I always welcome the worst cases, and this was certainly that kind of opportunity. However, I had no idea that one phone call would lead to my having four Upper Cervical clinics in Italy. This is the story of how that happened.

My mother-in-law, Ciadi, was born and grew up in Italy. She still has friends and family there who come to the states to visit her from time to time, so they were familiar with what I did as an Upper Cervical doctor. I adjusted Ciadi's brother and his wife when they came over, and Upper Cervical Care had helped them. That's probably why they called me about Damiana, a friend of theirs in Italy, whose husband had taken her to specialists in Italy, France, Germany, and Switzerland. Nobody knew what was wrong with Damiana or what to do for her. They just knew that what had been done had not helped; Damiana was getting worse instead of better.

When Damiana's symptoms were described to me, I said, "It sounds like dystonia." Dystonia is a neurological movement disorder in which involuntary muscle contractions cause twisting and repetitive movements or abnormal postures. This usually limits the patient's mobility, often to the point that the person suffering from dystonia can't function.

By the way, it is important to remember that the name of a particular disease is nothing more than a flowchart of symptoms. Someone decided that when these particular symptoms appear together, we're going to call it _____. (You can fill in the blank with any known disease.) That's why Upper Cervical doctors feel as comfortable adjusting a patient with multiple sclerosis as we do adjusting a patient with a headache. We don't claim to cure *anything*, but we *do* know that if a patient has nerve interference, it can manifest in the body in myriad ways. Those different "ways," take the form of various symptoms that have been labeled as particular diseases.

The World Health Organization has codes for all diseases that doctors use for diagnosis (and billing). In 2012 there were 14,199 such codes, which means there were 14,199 "billable diseases," and more are being added all the time.[32] A diagnosis is a doctor's best guess based on existing symptoms. Remember, doctors call their work a *practice,* not a sure thing. For some reason, it seems to help patients when they get a confirmed diagnosis. They now have a label for the symptoms they're experiencing. The downside is sometimes that label also brings fear, anxiety, or even hopelessness to the mind of the patient.

About a month after I had talked to Gianni, Damiana's husband, about Damiana's condition, a doctor in Switzerland told them that Damiana had dystonia. The fact that I had diagnosed her condition over the phone was enough to spark their interest, so they asked me if I could help her. I had, in fact, had several patients with dystonia who had done well under Upper Cervical Care. I also learned that Damiana had previously been diagnosed with cerebellar ataxia, and I had had a patient with cerebellar ataxia who had also responded well to Upper Cervical. Cerebellar ataxia is a motor disturbance; its symptoms include a patient's inability to coordinate balance, gait, and eye movement. I shared those experiences but reiterated that I didn't know how Damiana would respond to Upper Cervical Care.

When people ask me if Upper Cervical Care can help them, I can't promise them that it can. I can only share what I know. If I have worked with patients with the same condition who responded well under Upper Cervical Care, I tell them. If I have not worked with patients with their condition, I can only respond, "I don't know if Upper Cervical Care can help or not, but we should know within four to six weeks."

Damiana got a three-month visa, the maximum allowed, and came to Charlotte, North Carolina, to get under Upper Cervical Care. She was in a wheelchair, and her doctors had told Gianni that she would be dead in three months. After Damiana's first Upper Cervical adjustment, she slept through the night for the first time in a long time and woke up the next morning pain-free. Over time, her coordination improved. When she first came to me, her hand-to-eye coordination was very poor. Ciadi put an apple, a pencil, and a glass on a tray in front of Damiana and asked her to pick up the apple. Poor Damiana would knock everything else off the tray trying to pick up the apple. After Upper Cervical Care, Damiana could pick up the pencil with two fingers without disturbing any of the other items, a real feat for her.

When I first saw Damiana, her fingers were gnarled, and she had big knots on her joints. At the end of three months, these had cleared up. For me, the unforgettable moment came when Damiana got out of her wheelchair and walked, unassisted, down the hall of my clinic. (Damiana's story is detailed at the end of this chapter, and you can see a video of her progress under Upper Cervical Care by going to YouTube and typing "Damiana, upper cervical.")

Fortunately for me, Italians love to talk. Before Damiana got back to Italy, word had started to spread about this Upper Cervical doctor in America who had helped Damiana—who was supposed to be dead— come home pain-free and out of her wheelchair.

My next call from Italy came from two brothers, Antonio and Mario. Mario's four-year-old daughter, Dafne, was injured from a vaccine that caused swelling on her brain. Prior to the vaccination Dafne was a normal, healthy little girl; now she was paralyzed. When I got the call, doctors had told Mario his daughter would not live more than a few months. Her parents had been staying with Dafne in the pediatric hospital in Milan until the doctors sent Dafne home because there was nothing more they could do.

"Do you think Upper Cervical will help Dafne?" Mario asked. I could hear the hope in his voice.

"I don't know," I answered. "I move the bone. God does the healing. I don't know what kind of results Dafne will get from Upper Cervical Care. I do know that if we can improve the communication from the brain to her body, from the spiritual to the physical, from the creator to the created, her body will have the best chance it can possibly have to heal, to improve, to get her better."

Mario said all he wanted was to provide his daughter that chance.

I said, "Bring her over."

Within a few days, they arrived in Charlotte. Dafne's parents had spent all their savings on their daughter's medical treatments, so I treated Dafne *gratis*. After Dafne's very first Upper Cervical adjustment, her head, which had been leaning to one shoulder, was straight. Over the next three months, Dafne was able to feed herself, stand on her own, sleep through the night, control her bowels, and go to the bathroom. She was wearing diapers when she came to me. Dafne was here when she turned five, so we threw a little birthday party for her. I have her on video blowing me kisses. My two girls were about the same age, and they fell in love with Dafne. We all fell in love with Dafne. Dafne returned to Italy, greatly improved. (A video of Dafne can be found on YouTube by searching for "Dafne/uppercervical.")

Word continued to spread through Italy about Upper Cervical Care, and I continued to get calls. Now, I didn't want to go back into practice. I'd just left my practice to expand the Upper Cervical franchise, and I was committed to using my time, energy, and resources getting the word out about Upper Cervical here in the states. But I heard the pain and urgency in the voices over the phone; some told me if I would agree to see them I could "name my price."

Sixteen more patients came to see me from Italy. They came on a three-month visa, and I would see them after-hours, sometimes late at night, after I'd finished my work with Upper Cervical Health Centers. I had patients with ALS (Lou Gehrig's disease), fibromyalgia, Parkinson's, paralysis, and multiple sclerosis. Some patients, like Damiana and Dafne, had been given death sentences; all had debilitating conditions. And they all improved.

My Italian patients knew they would need follow-up care. They would need to be checked regularly to see if their adjustment was holding and to get adjusted again if it was not. That is the only way their healing would continue.

"How do we do that?" they began to ask. "Do we fly back to the states once a month? Do we fly you to Italy?"

"I guess either is a possibility," I replied.

"You know, Dr. Drury, look at how many people from Italy came here for Upper Cervical Care. Imagine if you had a practice in Italy. All the people who couldn't come here would come see you once they learned what Upper Cervical can do for them."

A doctor who was training with me at the time was listening. "I'd love to go open a practice for you in Italy," he said.

So I started thinking about it. I went to Italy and met with Damiana's husband, Gianni, who drove me around northern Italy, where they were from. In Italy, neither medical doctors nor chiropractors can take X-rays. That was a hurdle because Upper Cervical requires that we have very specific X-rays to determine if an adjustment is needed.

I opened my first clinic in Europe in the Republic of San Marino, one of the smallest republics in the world, and in the center of Italy, because San Marino did not have rules restricting the use of X-ray equipment. We could bring in our own X-ray machines and take our own X-rays.

"There is nothing more powerful than an idea whose time has come."

Victor Hugo

One day when I was demonstrating to some of the hospital personnel in San Marino the procedures Upper Cervical doctors use to determine if patients need to be corrected, I noticed a man and woman very attentively eavesdropping. After the demonstration, they came over and asked me to tell them more about how Upper Cervical works, which I did. I soon learned that the man, Antonio, had been diagnosed with ALS, Lou Gehrig's disease. What he and his wife really wanted to know is whether or not Upper Cervical Care could help Antonio.

By now, you know how I answered that. I told Antonio that I'd had other patients with Lou Gehrig's who had responded well to Upper Cervical Care, that all we do is move the bone that is interfering with the body's normal ability to heal, and that as long as there's no interference with the communication between the brain and the body, the body can adapt and heal itself.

I checked and scanned Antonio and showed him the blockage in the upper part of his neck that was interfering with the normal healing messages from his brain to his body. I explained that this blockage could be the cause of the symptoms he was experiencing that we label Lou Gehrig's disease. I told Antonio that he had the option of coming to the clinic in San Marino when it opened or coming to North Carolina with me. I had secured a space and negotiated a lease for my first Upper Cervical clinic in Europe and was headed back to the states. Antonio said he'd wait and go to the clinic in San Marino.

Four months later, Antonio's wife called me in Charlotte. "Dr. Drury, I need to bring Antonio to see you," she said.

I had just shipped everything we'd need to open the clinic in San Marino—X-ray equipment, scanners, tables, and computers. "We should be ready to open there in two months," I replied. "Just hang on." Then I heard crying on the other end.

"Dr. Drury, Antonio won't be here then. They've given him thirty days to live."

Antonio was in Charlotte the next day. When I first met Antonio in San Marino, he could talk and move himself around in the wheelchair. Now, four months later, Antonio could neither talk nor move his arms. He was paralyzed from head to toe.

"Antonio," I said when I saw him, "the first thing we have to do is to stop this thing from progressing. Now, you can't come over here and die on me because it's not going to look good when I go over there and open a clinic if you die on me here."

Antonio smiled faintly.

I continued to adjust Antonio until he began to hold the adjustment. Then Antonio started improving. He lived past the 30 days he was given to live; he lived past 60 days. He and his wife returned to Italy the day before my family and I left for Italy. When we had our office up and running in San Marino, Antonio continued his Upper Cervical Care. During the summer of 2012, I was in Italy visiting my clinics and in rolled Antonio and his wife, four years after he got his first Upper Cervical adjustment. Antonio was smiling. His wife was smiling. Heck, we were all smiling. Given 30 days to live, Antonio's not only still alive four years later, his health, and thus the quality of his life, has improved dramatically.

My first office in Italy was very successful. We had people from all over the country coming for Upper Cervical Care. Before long, our work began to attract the attention of some medical doctors there, but not in a negative way. They were interested in what we were doing and the results we were getting with Upper Cervical Care. Also, the hospitals in Italy wanted to know, as any business would, what we were doing that was attracting so many people.

I now have four Upper Cervical clinics in Europe. The one in San Marino has been moved to Rimini, Italy; the other three are in Rome, Sicily, and outside Venice. All four clinics are in hospitals. We trained the hospitals' X-ray technicians to take specific X-rays for our Upper Cervical doctors, and it has worked well. Europe has been a big part of the growth of Upper Cervical Health Centers, and we plan to expand into other parts of Europe as well as Asia.

I found a more level playing field in Italy, as doctors there are not controlled by the pharmaceutical industry. For example, when they hear about a study at the University of Chicago performed by *medical doctors* that proves that Upper Cervical Care reduces blood pressure equal to taking two blood pressure drugs at once, they're more than open to learning more about this procedure. In the United States, for whatever reason, that doesn't seem to happen. I'm hoping it's because not enough Americans know about Upper Cervical Care, and I'm also hoping this book will help change that.

I was introduced to Dr. Giuseppe Marceca, a vascular specialist in Rome, who wanted to know more about Upper Cervical. He knew Damiana and had seen how much she improved under Upper Cervical Care. Later that year, Dr. Marceca and Dr. Sandro Mandolesi, a medical doctor and friend and colleague of Dr. Marceca's, were present when I talked to TV and newspaper reporters in San Marino about Upper Cervical Care. I was surprised when Dr. Marceca stood up in front of his peers and the reporters and said that he had learned more in one hour with me than he had learned in all his years of medical school about how the body heals. He told the group gathered that although medicine is the best at diagnosis, it is not the best at helping people heal, and that medical doctors could learn a lot from the Upper Cervical doctor.

Dr. Marceca became so interested in Upper Cervical Care that he came to the states and spent a week visiting my clinics and talking to patients. Dr. Marceca began asking me, "Where is the research that shows how all these people are getting better? Where are the double-blind studies?"

I shared what I knew about the published Upper Cervical research and explained apologetically that because Upper Cervical doctors work independently in their individual offices, there is little collective research. I told Dr. Marceca that it was my goal to create an organization of Upper Cervical doctors which, in time, could afford to conduct the kind of research about which he spoke, research that we both understood was much needed. But right now, we're newly formed, I explained, and we don't have a lot of money to put into proving what we do. *We know what we do works because we see the results we get in our practices.*

"I understand," Dr. Marceca said, "but if you had scientific evidence, and the double-blind studies to prove it, the whole world would want what you have."

"Well," I replied, sighing, "we don't have it."

I remember that day in 2008 like it was yesterday. Dr. Marceca looked me in the eye and said, "Dr. Drury, I want to prove, scientifically, to the world what you know to be true clinically in your practice. I want to *scientifically* discover Upper Cervical Care."

"Dr. Marceca," I said, smiling, "have at it. We've been doing this for over one hundred years, and we haven't been discovered yet. We're all quiet little practices scattered around mostly the United States and Canada. Please, discover us."

Dr. Marceca did the first Upper Cervical double-blind study on multiple sclerosis, which you will read about in Chapter Nine. The ongoing research on Upper Cervical Care coming out of Italy is proving the science behind the healings—healings that Upper Cervical doctors have been witnessing for decades. Perhaps this new research will be the catalyst that brings Upper Cervical into the public's awareness, so it can help millions more.

***

Damiana, Upper Cervical Patient from Italy
Suffered from dystonia and cerebellar ataxia
(Interview done with the help of an interpreter)

Interpreter: *I met Damiana two months ago when I picked her up at the airport. She was in a wheelchair. She was doing really, really bad. I will have her explain to you how she felt.*

Damiana: *When I arrived in Charlotte, I was in a really bad stage. I was in so much pain. My hands were closed in clenched fists. I was all drawn up from the pain. After Upper Cervical adjustments, I am much more relaxed. He really helped me a lot. I'm no longer taking medications.*

After my first adjustment, the first night, I didn't have any pain through the night. I have been free of pain in my hand. Before, I was having a hard time to lift two fingers; they hurt so, so bad. But now I can open both hands and spread my fingers. It doesn't feel like it's real to me that I can open my hands. It's the first thing I do every morning is open my hands. I am so proud.

Now I'm able to do little things for myself. Before, I would reach for a glass, and I would shake really, really bad, but now I'm able to grab it with no problem.

Interpreter: *Also, when Damiana arrived in the states, I* *could barely understand her when she spoke. Her tongue went between her teeth and she had so much saliva that we were constantly having to wipe her mouth. Around her tenth day under Upper Cervical Care, her speech started getting much, much better. We don't have to wipe the saliva from her mouth anymore. She's doing really, really well.*

Damiana also told me that before the Upper Cervical adjustments, when someone asked her for a glass, she had to put into her mind what a glass looked like. On her third day, I brought a tray to her with 10 things on it. I started asking her to pick up the things as I called them out. As I asked for each item, Damiana would just go for the item, no shaking or anything, and pick it up and give it to me as soon as I asked for something. (Remember, she couldn't unclench her fist three days before.) To me, it was a miracle. It really was.

She is so proud of everything because she told me when she was in Italy that she was just waiting to die. The doctors had told her there was nothing else that could be done for her. At 50, she was only waiting to die. In two months, I have seen her, both mentally and physically, improve 100% to me.

NOTE: Watch the YouTube video titled "Damiana—Upper Cervical Care" to see Damiana walking down the hall of my Upper Cervical office, two months after arriving in the United States in a wheelchair. Love that smile. You'll understand what I mean when you watch it. Words can't explain.

The day we shot the video on Damiana my waiting room happened to be full of patients from Italy who had come over for Upper Cervical Care. The beautiful little girl you hear me call the Hollywood star is Dafne whom I wrote about in this chapter. After Upper Cervical Care, Dafne was able to hold her head up, sit up, feed herself, stand for short periods of time, and blow me kisses, none of which she was able to do prior to Upper Cervical Care. View her YouTube video, "Think Twice About Vaccinations—Dafne," but be prepared to have your heart hurt.

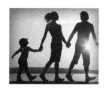

CHAPTER 7

Upper Cervical Care for Children

"It is easier to build strong children than to repair broken men."

Frederick Douglass

I'm going to answer the two questions you're probably already asking: (1) Should children be under chiropractic care? The answer is yes, absolutely, and (2) Is chiropractic care safe for children? The answer is, again, yes, absolutely. As Upper Cervical doctor and pediatric diplomate Dr. Julie Mayer Hunt puts it: When do you get kids' teeth checked? When they have them. When do you get their spine checked? When they have one.

Let's deal with the safety issue first. A 2009 study by the International Chiropractic Pediatric Association (ICPA) on 577 children under chiropractic care showed that doctors reported only three adverse events, minor discomfort after the adjustment, which was readily resolved with continued adjustments. All children remained under chiropractic care, and both parents and doctors indicated a high rate of improvement with respect to the children presenting complaints. In addition to these improvements, respondents reported better sleeping patterns in their children, improvements in their behavior, and improved immune system function while their children were under chiropractic care.[33]

Our two daughters have been under Upper Cervical Care since birth, and I would *never* subject them to anything that wasn't both safe and beneficial. They're in first and second grade now, and at the end of the last school year, the kindergarten teacher who had both our girls said to my wife, "Your kids are the healthiest I've ever taught." The teacher, pregnant with her first child, wanted to know what we did to keep our kids healthy so she could do the same thing for her child. You can guess what our answer was.

Upper Cervical doctors love working with little ones; children respond so quickly. I remember one of my little patients, who I saw during my first year in practice. Chelsea was 18 months old and having epileptic seizures. Sometimes her mother would bring her in, and sometimes the babysitter. When I first saw Chelsea, she was lethargic and unresponsive, perhaps because this little toddler was on three different high-powered medications.

I remember the day Chelsea's babysitter called me crying and panicked. She told me she had held the cap of one of the medicine bottles between her teeth while she used a syringe to give Chelsea her medication. Moments later, the babysitter's face went numb from the tiny bit of medication that got on her lip while she was holding the bottle cap in her mouth.

"I can't imagine what this medicine is doing to her little body if it did that to me!" the babysitter cried.

I could only agree that little Chelsea had been pre-scribed some powerful meds.

Under Upper Cervical Care, Chelsea's seizures began to taper off, and her mother started weaning her daughter off the meds. Within four months, the child who had been brought into my office zombie-like was off all her medication; the seizures had stopped, and Chelsea had blossomed into this beautiful, active little girl with an engaging personality, interacting with my office staff and making us Valentine cards. Awesome to witness.

Dr. Julie Mayer Hunt remembers the 20-month-old who, when he was brought to her office, had never had a bowel movement on his own. Not only was the little boy miserable, his parents were so stressed they were con-sidering divorce. This little boy had already had lumbar spinal surgery. Doctors said he wasn't pooping because he had anal stenosis, so they used an anal dilator on him. One of his legs was shorter than the other, and the whole lumbar spine was contracted on one side. Dr. Mayer Hunt helped get the toddler balanced the way his body was designed to work. Over a two-month period, the little boy was off his medication and having regular bowel move-ments. He's now a normal, healthy child who, Dr. Mayer Hunt believes, never needed surgery. His parents, who were about to break up when they brought their son in for Upper Cervical Care, are still together, and at the time Dr. Mayer Hunt related this story, they were expecting their second child.

Sometimes the recoveries children make astound us. Dr. Thad Vuagniaux remembers the seven-year-old deaf girl we have on video from the mission trip a group of Upper

Cervical doctors made to Moldova of the former Soviet Republic. The little girl looked so timid and scared as the interpreter tried to reassure her. After she got adjusted, the little girl got up and looked around at the hundreds of people talking and moving about in the noisy auditorium. Then she grabbed her ears and started screaming. Her hearing had been restored.

Often, after adult patients have been helped by Upper Cervical Care, they start asking if Upper Cervical can help their children. This was the case with Lauren, a 16-month-old whose mother's neck and back pain had gone away under Upper Cervical Care. Lauren was born prematurely and had never used her right hand and arm. Lauren's pediatric neurologist told her mother that Lauren might never have the use of her arm. After her first Upper Cervical adjustment, Lauren began to use her arm, and within a few weeks, no one could tell she'd ever had a problem with it. On Lauren's last visit to the pediatric neurologist, the neurologist said everything looked great and that sometimes, for no known reason, these things can heal.

Lauren had been sick since birth with constant colds, a runny nose, cough, and fever. She rarely slept more than a few hours. Her poor health, plus having been poked and prodded by doctors her whole life, resulted in her being very difficult to check and adjust. She fought her parents and me, kicking and screaming, from the moment she arrived until she was post-checked and left the office. The second time I saw Lauren, the runny nose, coughing, and fever had cleared up, and her mom said she had been sleeping much better. But, here's the coolest part: When I went to check Lauren this time, this little 16-month-old baby girl looked up at me, then bent her head indicating she was ready for me to check her. Then she climbed up on the table and assumed the position for me to adjust her. Her dad said, "Holy cow, do you think she knows that this is good for her?"

After I adjusted her, Lauren stood up, looked at us with a big smile, took a deep breath, and exhaled with an audible sigh as if to say, "Oh! That's what I needed." We all looked at each other in amazement.

Another patient whom I'll never forget was Amanda. Amanda's mother was eager to get help for her daughter and reluctantly shared that Amanda had been a victim of shaken baby syndrome, which she thought might be the reason Amanda had seizures—now multiple seizures, daily. Not only did Amanda's seizures go away under Upper Cervical Care, that 10-year-old is now in chiropractic school. Amanda will, of course, be an Upper Cervical doctor.

Again, it's usually the parents who come to Upper Cervical for care; later, they bring in their kids. Amanda's story was the other way around. A few years ago, Amanda's mother stood up at a meeting I had to introduce more people to Upper Cervical Care. I was sure she was going to tell Amanda's story when she stood up, but she surprised me.

"Dr. Drury doesn't even know the full story I'm going to tell you," Amanda's mother began. "A few years ago, I was diagnosed with COPD (chronic obstructive pulmonary disease). The doctor showed me the X-rays. I had several large masses on my lungs, and the doctors told me I wouldn't live much longer. I was a single mom raising two young girls. Amanda was the youngest and was having several grand mal seizures every day. I knew I had to get her help before I left her without a mother. Someone at church told me Dr. Drury had helped people who had seizures. I took Amanda and her seizures did get better. When I saw how well Amanda was doing, I decided to see Dr. Drury myself. Six months later, I went back to my pulmonologist. They took new X-rays, and they were clear. No masses! No COPD!"

"You never know how far-reaching something you may say, think, or do today may affect the lives of millions tomorrow."

B. J. Palmer

The prejudice against chiropractic care for adults pales when compared to the prejudice against chiropractic care for children. Dr. Daniel Kuhn, a beloved and highly respected Upper Cervical doctor who went to Palmer College when B. J. Palmer was there, illustrates this with an example from his own practice.

"I worked with an incredible couple," Dr. Kuhn said, "who had six cribs in their home for babies who couldn't walk. These children were in foster care. If these babies learned to walk, they would be moved to other caregivers; that was the arrangement this couple had with the state. They had hydrocephalus, cerebral palsy, convulsions, all kinds of things going on; they were children that had been given up on, basically. Every time the foster parents of these special-needs children got a new child, they would immediately bring that child into our office for Upper Cervical Care. Well, so many of them started getting better that the social worker said to these foster parents, 'I don't know what they're doing, but the doctors you're taking these kids to are miracle workers.' The foster parents were afraid to tell the social worker that they were taking these children to a chiropractor because they were afraid if they did, they'd lose their license. That's a sad but true story."

I wish in this chapter I could just write about what a great wellness program Upper Cervical Care is for children, but unfortunately, just like adults, kids do get sick. A growing body of research shows how Upper Cervical Care is helping children of all ages regain health and vitality, allowing them to be happy, active kids again.

Parents, please educate yourself about the drugs that are being prescribed to your children. Reuters reported in 2002 that kids had surpassed senior citizens as the "hot ticket for prescription drugs," with the number of prescriptions for children increasing 85% in five years.[34] In June, 2012, *Health Day News* reported that the number of prescriptions written for children had dropped by 7%. So prescriptions written for children have increased only 78% in the last 20 years. We should be happy about this? (By the way, the number of prescriptions written for adults have *increased* by 22% over the last 10 years, according to the same report.)

"The best doctor gives the least medicine."

Benjamin Franklin

The reasons given for the 7% decrease in prescriptions written for children were that several of the allergy-medication prescriptions are now available over-the-counter; the black-box warnings that have been added to depression medication drugs describing an increased risk of suicide may have led to a decrease in prescriptions for children; and finally, a decrease in the number of antibiotic prescriptions for children might be consistent with efforts to decrease the risk of antibiotic resistance. (Parents, please hear me: Viruses, such as the common cold, do *not* respond to antibiotics.) However, in the last 10 years there has been an *increase* in the number of drugs written for children in three categories—prescriptions for asthma, ADHD, and contraceptives.[35]

The value of appropriate medications for serious conditions is recognized, but again, parents need to question the necessity, efficacy, and safety of all prescription drugs. Studies show that children who took antibiotics during infancy had a fourfold risk of developing asthma.[36]

Parents must also recognize the power of their influence. If we give even a subtle or implicit message to our children that when you feel bad, you take a pill, should we be all that surprised when, as adolescents, our children turn to recreational drugs when they want to feel good? What if they were taught as children that health comes from within, not without, that the body has the ability to heal itself? Wouldn't having our children know and live this truth go a long way toward ensuring they live a healthier life as children and later, as adults?

Some people look at me funny when I tell them that infants should have their Upper Cervical area checked

for a subluxation as soon as possible. Trauma to the upper cervical area can occur during the birth process even
in controlled settings. During labor, the spinal column,
especially the cervical portion, may be injured if the fetus
is compressed and forced down the birth canal.

There is research to support this. Dr. Ludwig Gutmann,
a German medical doctor, observed that 80% of his infant patients had an atlas blockage, a type of vertebral
subluxation. The paper he published on this clearly cor-
relates structural dysfunction with neurological interference. Gutmann found that radiographic (X-ray) analysis
was of decisive importance, and the intervention he described appears to be a typical chiropractic adjustment.
These findings were echoed in the case studies of another
German doctor, Dr. Biedermann, who asserted that radiographic analysis is the key to a successful upper cervical
adjustment.[37]

I will summarize some of the research that supports the
effectiveness of Upper Cervical Care in treating conditions
normally associated with children, this time listing them
in the approximate order they might occur, starting with
infancy. (For those who would like a more detailed, clinical explanation of these studies, I refer you to Dr. Kirk
Eriksen's book, *Upper Cervical Subluxation Complex:
A Review of the Chiropractic and Medical Literature*.)

Breast-feeding difficulties: Upper Cervical corrections
resulted in the restoration of natural suckling patterns for
two infants ranging in age from two days to four months.[38]

Infantile colic: Infantile colic may not be a life-threat-
ening condition, but it can be extremely stressful to the

baby and parents. In a study published in the *Journal of Manipulative and Physiological Therapeutics*, of 316 infants suffering from colic, 94% of the babies receiving an Upper Cervical correction had a successful outcome.[39]

In a study done by the Danish National Health Service, 50 babies with infantile colic were randomly placed in two groups. One group of 25 was given a drug treatment (Dimethicone) for their colic; the other group was placed under chiropractic care. At the end of two weeks, the crying from infants under chiropractic care had reduced an average of 3.9 hours per day. The crying from infants on Dimethicone had reduced by an average of one hour per day. All 25 of the babies under chiropractic care stayed in the study the full 13 days, and five of the babies given the drug treatment did not complete the study. When contacted, three of the parents of the babies who dropped out of the study said they did so because their baby's colic had worsened, instead of improved, with the drug.[40]

SIDS: Sudden infant death syndrome, or SIDS, is the sudden, unexplained death of a baby under one year old. It is the most common cause of infant death in developed countries and affects close to 3,000 babies each year in the United States alone. The incidence of SIDS peaks at two to four months, with 95% of the cases occurring prior to the time a baby is six months old. The cause of sudden infant death syndrome has been attributed to many conditions. Upper cervical dysfunction and instability should be added to the list.

There is compelling evidence that a brain stem-SIDS correlation exists. Both medical and chiropractic researchers have suggested the relationship between SIDS and the brain stem, spinal cord, or upper cervical area. More than 100 research studies point to the brain stem as a critical link to SIDS. Researchers J. Lucena and F.F. Cruz-Sánchez stated, "Brain stem dysfunction of circuits that control respiration and cardiovascular stability may be involved in SIDS. It is postulated that this abnormality originates in utero and leads to sudden death during a vulnerable postnatal period."[41]

In an article in *Human Spine in Health and Disease,* SIDS is discussed as possibly being the result of birth trauma, cervical subluxation, and subsequent brain stem involvement. Another article in *Forensic Science International* discusses a hypothesis that explains how mechanical irritation of the upper cervical region can serve as a trigger that may be involved in SIDS. This investigation involved 695 infants between the ages of one month and a year old.[42]

The challenge we have with SIDS and doing research to suggest a preventative value from chiropractic treatment is that SIDS is a diagnosis that is only made after the death of an infant, and, therefore, it is nearly impossible to prove prevention. However, Dr. Ronald Harper and his team at UCLA found instances of abnormal respiratory control in infants who later died of SIDS, and Upper Cervical chiropractors have seen children who had difficulty breathing have their breathing normalize after an Upper Cervical correction. Also, since the medical research suggests the brain stem is associated with SIDS, and the purpose of an Upper Cervical correction is to remove nerve interference in this area, it is highly probable that children under Upper Cervical Care are less likely to succumb to SIDS.[43]

Ear Infections (otis media): The standard medical approach to treating an ear infection is administering antibiotics and surgery (implementation of tubes). The problems with antibiotics include allergic reactions, gastrointestinal upset, destruction of intestinal flora, yeast infection, drug resistance, cost, and the fact that they are often not effective. Scientific evidence has shown that the indiscriminate use of antibiotics and surgical implementation of tubes is usually not effective. Dr. J. O. Hendley, a pediatrician from the University of Virginia, wrote an article in the *New England Journal of Medicine* in which he stated that antibiotics help only one in eight children with ear infections. Tympanostomy tubes treat the symptoms, not the cause of the problem.[44] Upper Cervical doctors report successfully treating children with ear infections and perhaps more importantly, report that children under regular Upper Cervical Care rarely *get* ear infections.

Autism: Autism is a vaguely defined neurodevelopmental disorder. Symptoms can range from violence to withdrawn behavior. The incidence of autism has skyrocketed in the past 20 years, as it previously affected about one in 10,000 children. In 1997, the United States Centers for Disease Control, the CDC, estimated that autism affected one in 500.[45] The CDC's 2012 estimate is one in 88 children are diagnosed with autism every year, a 78% increase since 2007. Four times as many boys have autism as girls.[46]

Leading authorities in the field of autism believe, and neurophysiologic experiments suggest, that the brain stem is involved in autism, and that dysfunction of the specific neural network that accounts for the behavioral syndrome of autism may be due to a wide variety of insults to the developing brain.[47] Upper Cervical doctors believe this may explain the success they have had working with children who have the symptoms of autism.

ADD and ADHD: The number of children diagnosed with ADD (attention deficit disorder) and ADHD (attention deficit hyperactivity disorder) has skyrocketed in the last 15 to 20 years. These disorders tend to affect boys two to three times as frequently as girls. Children may get labeled ADHD if they exhibit these characteristics: distractibility, impulsivity, and hyperactivity. The problem is most children exhibit at least some of these behaviors. Knowing this, in 1994, the American Academy of Pediatrics created diagnostic criteria for ADHD that included two sets of nine specific symptoms and behaviors. The child must display at least six of the nine symptoms and behaviors, and the manifestations must have persisted for at least six months to a degree that is maladaptive and inconsistent with the child's developmental level. The problem is the assessment requires evidence directly obtained from parents, caregivers, and classroom teachers regarding the core symptoms as they relate to various settings, age of onset, duration of symptoms, and degree of functional impairment. However, due to time constraints and other pressures, such a thorough evaluation is seldom done.[48]

What is more frequently done is that the child is prescribed a stimulant medication such as methylphenidate (Ritalin). The rate of medication used for these disorders has doubled every two to four years since 1971. Ritalin, a drug that an estimated six million children in the United States take daily, is a Class II drug, in the same category as cocaine, methadone, methamphetamine, and opium. The United States consumes about 90% of all the Ritalin produced worldwide.[49]

Peter R. Breggin, MD, Director of the International Center for the Study of Psychiatry and Psychology and associate faculty member at Johns Hopkins University Department of Counseling stated, "Ritalin does not correct biochemical imbalances—it causes them." Dr. Breggin also indicated that methylphenidate can cause depression, agitation, social withdrawal, and a decreased ability to learn.[50]

Early childhood is a pivotal period in the development of the human brain. *The Physicians' Desk Reference* (PDR), 50th Edition, notes that methylphenidate should not be administered to children under age six since safety and efficacy for this age group have not been established. (Long-term use of this drug in terms of safety and efficacy has not been established for children of any age.) The PDR goes on to list 23 possible side effects for children taking methylphenidate including worsening of behavior, disturbances of thought disorders, drug dependence, anorexia, psychotic episodes, and Tourette syndrome.[51]

To me, it's unconscionable that we're putting so many children on such a high-powered drug, and what's more unbelievable is that we're doing this when there is little evidence of long-term benefits to children with ADHD who take these medications. No difference has been found between chemically treated and untreated ADHD patients in terms of failed grades, achievement scores, memory retention, or anger control. Another study found that after eight years of stimulant medication, 80% of the children continue to have ADHD symptoms.[52]

Upper Cervical Care is an option that should be explored for children suffering from the symptoms of ADD or ADHD. My colleagues and I have successfully worked with children exhibiting the symptoms of ADD and ADHD. Upper Cervical doctors do not treat ADHD or any other condition, as I've stated many times. Instead, we focus on finding and removing a subluxation that might be putting stress on the nervous system. When that stress is removed, it improves the neurological integrity and allows the body to start healing itself, as it was created to do.

"After children have had an Upper Cervical adjustment, you can literally see their expressions change. They go from cranky and fussy to 'the light is on.'"

Dr. Daniel Kuhn, Upper Cervical Chiropractor

Scoliosis: Scoliosis is a condition in which the spine bends to the side abnormally, either to the left or to the right. Several studies correlate pelvic distortion with scoliosis. Spinal curves, particularly double curvatures, can increase as children go through preadolescence and adolescent growth spurts. One study showed that when screening was done by X-ray, two-thirds of the girls had mild scoliosis. An increase in the scoliotic curve(s) of five degrees over a three-month period is considered a rapid advancement in scoliosis, and such cases should be closely monitored. In one case study, a nine-year-old boy with juvenile idiopathic scoliosis and intermittent back pain, had an 88% overall reduction after five months under Upper Cervical Care.[53]

In addition, corrective spinal surgery is usually only indicated in patients whose curves have advanced to over 40 degrees, and then, the long-term benefits of spinal surgery for scoliosis correction are debatable.[54] It just seems logical that a doctor of chiropractic who is trained to work exclusively with the spine would be the specialist to examine children with scoliosis before such drastic treatments are considered.

According to the American Chiropractic Association, the number of children under chiropractic care has risen 8.5% since 1991. When surveyed by the International Chiropractic Pediatric Association (ICPA), parents reported that under chiropractic care, they saw improvement in their children's behavior, their children slept better, and their children had a stronger immune system.[55]

Sometimes, Upper Cervical Care can return to a child the life he thought he had lost, like it did for David. His story is next.

Julia, Mother of David S., Upper Cervical Patient
Suffered from multiple debilitating symptoms following an injury

Near the end of sixth grade, David banged his head against a wall while playing basketball. Fearing he might have suffered a concussion, his dad and I took him to an Urgent Care Center. They told us to wake David up every three hours that night, which we did. Everything seemed okay.

However, shortly after the accident, we noticed changes in David. His agility wasn't as good; this is a kid who'd been very athletic, but now he wasn't as flexible. Plus, his attitude seemed to change without provocation. But because David was approaching puberty, the family wrote off the change in his behavior to middle school madness and the awkwardness of a changing body.

Then the seizures started, so we took David to what became a long list of specialists. After several doctors, two MRIs, four high-powered medications, and a nerve conductive study revealed nothing unusual, a neurologist suggested David's condition was psychosomatic, that David was making this up to get attention.

That was one of the most frustrating things we, as parents, had to deal with. Instead of looking at David's symptoms and asking what could be the cause, the medical doctors decided the kid had to be faking it. It was a simple case of "You don't fit in a box that I know, so I'm not going to look any further." What they do instead is refer you, refer you, and refer you, and each specialist looks only at his particular body part. I think in medicine you must be taught that you can't say you don't know, so you steamroll ahead. All we knew was David wasn't getting any better, and we were getting poorer. The doctor bills just kept coming.

This was such a stressful time for the whole family; everything revolved around David's condition. It was especially hard on David's relationship with his dad, who began to wonder if David was faking it, and David knew his father was beginning to doubt him. That's heartbreaking, and very divisive. Plus, our younger daughter was pretty much on her own. She didn't get the attention she deserved. We just lived in crisis mode.

After one seizure, they did an MRI and the doctor called us and told us it was normal. Then about a week after those results, David had a seizure in his pediatrician's office. The pediatrician was shocked. He went back and read the MRI report. There were three boxes on the MRI that could be checked: Normal, Abnormal, and Inconclusive. Inconclusive is the box that was checked. It said, "Evidence of swelling at the base of the skull. We recommend further study of the base." But because it wasn't the brain, the neurologist said the results were normal. This is how things happen, and we had no clue because we didn't get a copy of the MRI report.

When the neurologist told us the brain scan was normal, that made us think that maybe he was right, maybe David was making this up. I'm sure this neurologist is very good with someone who has a tumor or an obvious brain injury from, say, a car wreck, but David didn't fit into his box. He gave David a prescription and told us to come back in six weeks.

I felt that some of the doctors who saw David didn't really care. I mean, you have a 20-minute appointment. Each time, you have to explain what's going on, who you've seen, the medications you've taken; you leave with nothing new, except maybe another prescription.

Here's an example: Once, a doctor we trusted finally told us that he didn't know what was going on with David, *but there had to be someone in our city who did. He told us to go to the emergency room and to sit there until somebody saw David, which we did, for six hours. The only thing we got from our visit to the emergency room was a $6,000 bill for tests, some of which David had already had, so the insurance company wouldn't pay. How does a patient know which tests doctors have done? You don't even know what's covered and what's not covered until the bills come in. We also learned that you are charged for the examining room by the hour and that if you're in the hospital during meal time, you get charged for meals, even if you never see a meal, which David didn't. It's crazy. Where's the caring, the compassion? You're just at the mercy of the system.*

David continued to have seizures. He couldn't walk because his brain couldn't tell his body how. It wasn't that he couldn't physically walk; his brain just wasn't communicating with his body. We found that if we started moving his legs we could get him to kind of drag across the room. We started researching wheelchairs for David. He was now experiencing tremors and involuntary movements in both hands. One time his hand struck the table so violently he broke his wrist.

At this point, we couldn't leave him alone. David couldn't go to school. He had such bad headaches that he couldn't read, so we listened to books on tape. Basically, David lay on the floor, and we put quilts around him, so if he started hitting things, he couldn't do much damage. Depression set in, and David started gaining weight because he couldn't do anything. Doctors just kept sending him home with a prescription and telling us to come back in six weeks. I'm sorry, but that's not what a parent wants to hear.

Finally, our pediatrician sent us to a neurologist at Duke. We took a video of David having a seizure, so the doctors could see for themselves. So many times in the past David would be fine in the doctor's office, and once we were in the car to come home, he'd start flailing about. The neurologist at Duke was honest to admit he didn't know what could be causing the seizures David was having, but he discounted the idea that they were psychosomatic, which made David feel better.

One day when I was picking up a prescription for David, I ran into Sonja Drury, David's first-grade teacher. We started chatting about David, and she suggested I take David to see her husband, who is an Upper Cervical chiropractor. Well, I didn't know anything about Upper Cervical, but we had taken David to a general chiropractor, and not only did it not help, David said the adjustment hurt and he didn't want to go back, so we didn't.

But I trusted Sonja, and we were desperate. I remember the day her husband first saw David. He said, "I have good news and bad news. David does have a problem, but it's fixable." Now, I'm not a medical person, but when the doctor put David's X-ray up on the screen, I saw what he was pointing out to us, and it sounded right to me. He explained David's atlas was badly out of alignment, probably as a result of the injury he had playing basketball when he was in the sixth grade. He used a model and drawings to show us exactly what he would be doing, and that raised my comfort level.

David saw the Upper Cervical doctor every day until he could hold an adjustment. I compare it to a blister where the atlas bone is rubbing on the brain stem. That's why it took so long and there's a progression. It had to heal, and it took time. You can't speed up the healing; all you can do is support it. It was about two weeks before we started seeing improvement. Our first Upper Cervical appointment was right after Thanksgiving in 2008, and David's last seizure was the 23rd of December, about a month later. In the middle of January, David started back to school.

Upper Cervical is the only thing we found in three years of searching, searching, searching, that helped David get well. When we went back to the neurologist at Duke, I told him how David had been helped by Upper Cervical. The neurologist said, "You know, I think we can learn from each other how the body works, and there are different times when different things work." I thought that was good. He didn't come from the stance of "Western medicine is good, chiropractic is bad," so maybe things are changing. When we had first told David's pediatrician that we were taking David to an Upper Cervical chiropractor, he said, "You're doing what?" But when he saw the turnaround David made, he was impressed.

We incurred over $50,000 of debt trying to find help for David, and we had insurance! But they would do these tests, then the insurance wouldn't pay because there wasn't a diagnosis. It was mind-boggling. If you don't have a label for your condition, then they just deny that you have anything wrong with you. If you can't say what it is, it must be in your head. It's crazy. But the body is *this amazing organism, and it does things we don't know about—without our permission or knowing, it tries to fix itself. And when you have things like seizures, that's a warning that something's off.*

What I think Upper Cervical does is give people a framework that makes sense. Upper Cervical starts with the premise that the body's connected, and David had a bad connection. If it were a house we were talking about, and you said the wiring got exposed and we have to cover the wiring, people would get it.

Don't insurance companies know they could save a ton of money if they started paying more for preventive care like Upper Cervical? Prevention has to be cheaper than drugs and surgery.

It took awhile before David could hold the adjustment, but now he's holding them really well. It's been a long time now since he's had to be adjusted. David's doing great. He's a sophomore in high school, in an International Baccalaureate program. Right now, he's working on a project based on his experience. He wants his peers to know that a head or neck injury can lead to debilitating conditions in other parts of the body. David said he doesn't want anyone to have to go through what he went through.

For three years, we lived this nightmare around David's mysterious illness. Now life is getting back to normal for all of us. David recently eagled in Boy Scouts. He's so happy to have his life back. We all are.

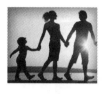

CHAPTER 8

From Quacks to Facts

"It's difficult to get someone to understand something when his salary depends upon his not understanding it."

Upton Sinclair

Since chiropractic came into being in 1895, it has had its dissenters, and history shows that most of them have come from the medical profession. The life of a medical doctor was vastly different then than it is today. Medicine was just emerging as a profession with licensures, codes of conduct, and required studies at medical schools, which began to proliferate during the mid-1800's. At that time, the role of the doctor did not have a clear class position, as there was a lot of inequality. Doctors did not earn much, and a physician's status depended largely on his family's status.[56] There was no American Medical Association to look out for doctors' interests, no insurance companies to ensure them a steady stream of patients, and no billion-dollar pharmaceutical manufacturers with a vested interest in their success.

It is understandable that the medical community would look at this new, unproven practice called chiropractic with skepticism. After all, the Palmer School was seeing thousands of patients a week in its clinic. People came from all over the country for chiropractic treatment, and they kept coming because they were being helped. B. J. Palmer was never shy about promoting chiropractic; he published volumes of research and owned and operated two radio stations and a TV station to help validate the new profession.

It is recorded that when Dr. Charles Mayo brought his wife to the Palmer Clinic for Upper Cervical Care that he brought with him a huge file on her condition that he threw on the table in front of Dr. B. J. Palmer, which B. J. ignored.

"Don't you want to see her medical history, the tests and treatments she's had?" Dr. Mayo asked.

"No," B. J. replied.

"But my wife has been to some of the finest doctors in the United States and Europe," Dr. Mayo argued.

"And if what they did had worked, you wouldn't be here," Dr. Palmer answered.

Dr. Mayo watched as Dr. Palmer X-rayed his wife's spine, performed readings with the neurocalometer and neurocalograph, and gave her an upper cervical adjustment. B. J. said that he didn't know what was wrong with Mrs. Mayo, and he didn't have to know. Perhaps she did have osteochondromatosis of the knee joint as her medical doctors had diagnosed. B. J. explained that he knew Dr. Mayo's wife had a subluxation, which, according to chiropractic, was the *cause* of her illness because it was blocking her nervous system.

During their heated discussion, Dr. Mayo reportedly called Dr. B. J. Palmer ignorant while Dr. Palmer explained to Dr. Mayo that while the medical profession is concerned with learning everything it can about *effects* and primarily treating symptoms through drugs or surgery, chiropractic is concerned with locating and removing subluxations in the spine, which it believes to be the *cause* of disease.

Dr. Mayo said that if giving his wife an adjustment was all Dr. Palmer was going to do for his wife that it would be impossible for her to get well. But when Mrs. Mayo left the Palmer Clinic a few months later, Dr. Mayo admitted that he didn't know how what Dr. Palmer had done worked, but he had to acknowledge that it had. His wife was well.[57]

I relate the details of this story because I think it points to a primary reason the medical profession has denigrated chiropractic for most of its existence: They don't understand it, and sometimes it's easier to discount something you don't understand than it is to try to understand it.

We can all acknowledge that it's often not easy to accept new ideas, new ways of doing things, especially if those new ways run counter to what we've been taught to believe—and many people have been taught to believe that drugs and surgery are the only ways to restore health. Many of us have been programmed to accept that as truth, but it's time we accept that maybe it's not as true as we've been led to believe, or, at the very least, that maybe it's not true all the time for all people.

There was a time when 16% of all women who gave birth died from puerperal sepsis, or childbed fever. We now know these deaths were the result of infections caused by the bacteria introduced by the unclean hands of physicians. Dr. Ignaz Semmelweis, an obstetrician at Vienna General Hospital in 1846, discovered that he could reduce the mortality rate of his maternity patients to only 1% by simply washing his hands. He tried to proclaim this discovery to the world but was regarded as a quack among his colleagues, and his teachings were disregarded. When he provided overwhelming proof in his book, *The Etiology, Concept, and Prophylaxis of Childhood Fever,* he provoked even greater hostility among his medical contemporaries. In 1865, Dr. Semmelweis was tricked by jealous colleagues into visiting a mental asylum. When he tried to leave the asylum, he was forcibly restrained. Semmelweis died in that asylum, and not until several years after his death did the medical community become convinced of the validity of his discovery, and all doctors began routinely washing their hands before delivering babies.[58] It is not particularly surprising then, that the chiropractic approach to health care has taken time to gain acceptance.

In the 1950s if there was negativity toward chiropractic, it was based on the belief that it was a young, upstart profession that was yet to be scientifically proven. However, chiropractors were getting excellent results, and it was generally believed that public knowledge would catch up with what doctors of chiropractic knew to be true. During this time, some chiropractors developed professional relationships with medical doctors in terms of both communication and patient referrals. There was a growing mutual respect and cooperation between the professions.

However, in the early 1960s, all that changed. When chiropractic was beginning to experience a surge of public popularity, an onslaught of published material maligning chiropractic started circulating, which had a devastating effect on the profession. It seemed that the more successes chiropractic had with patients, clinical studies, and professional development, the more outlandish and offensive the attacks against chiropractic. By the late '60s, the attacks had become so pervasive and vicious that it became clear that the underlying intent was to create public fear and distrust of the chiropractic profession.

Articles attacking chiropractic appeared in newspapers, magazines, and newsletters all over the country. Expressions like "unscientific cult" were used to refer to chiropractors. These publications began to echo each other, using the same catchphrases over and over. It was becoming obvious that the similarities in the attacks were in no way coincidental.

Chiropractors were appalled at the attacks and the inaccuracies being circulated, often in national publications, but they really didn't know how to fight back. Angry and frustrated, some wrote articles in protest, but these were primarily published in chiropractic journals and not read by the general public. Most chiropractors quietly continued in their practices, helping sick people get well, in the midst of all the negative propaganda.

Needless to say, the progress made in the way the medical and chiropractic professions worked together in the 1950s had all but reversed by the mid-1960s, as MDs were told not to refer patients to chiropractors or to associate with chiropractors professionally. Outlandish claims meant to discredit chiropractic continued to circulate, including one that said in 1945 *Medical World News* reported one could order a degree in chiropractic from a college in Chicago for $127.50. However, when contacted, the librarian of that publication could find no record of such a claim ever being made in *Medical World News*, which was not even published until 1960!

After a time, internal documents and memos surfaced that revealed that none other than the American Medical Association was publishing and distributing the anti-chiropractic propaganda. Unfortunately, readers tend to believe the printed word, especially when it comes from an organization like the AMA, an organization that we've been taught is there to protect and enlighten us, an organization that has both wealth and public support.

However, the truth is, the AMA is nothing more than a private trade organization representing the collective interests of its members, those who work in the field of medicine. The AMA was, and still is, one of the most powerful lobbying groups in the nation.

Why would a prestigious and powerful organization like the AMA go after chiropractors?

Possible reasons include: (1) Chiropractic was getting results and therefore growing in popularity and acceptance; (2) Chiropractic doesn't prescribe drugs, so pharmaceutical companies have nothing to gain, and perhaps much to lose, if people went to chiropractors instead of medical doctors; and (3) They didn't want chiropractors to be paid by insurance companies or be covered under Medicare. More internal documents from within the AMA surfaced that revealed the AMA was deeply concerned about competition from chiropractors.

In addition to publishing slanderous and erroneous information about chiropractic in various national

publications, the AMA's campaign to discredit and eliminate chiropractors also included: (1) Organizing and fund-
ing a committee it called the Committee on Quackery;
they first called it the Committee on Chiropractic, then
changed it to the more negative terminology to make it
appear their efforts were intended to save the public from
a bunch of quacks; and (2) Organizing a boycott preventing
association by any of its members with anyone representing chiropractic interests or services and enlisting the
support of other groups including the Joint Commission,
which accredits hospitals. Therefore, hospitals stopped
associating with chiropractors in fear they would lose their
accreditation.

On October 17, 1974, chiropractors and supporters of
chiropractic from five states came together to form the
National Chiropractic Antitrust Committee (NCAC) to
bring charges against the AMA for violating the United
States anitrust laws. The Clayton Act of 1914 made monopolies that prevent free competition illegal.

An informant inside the AMA, who identified himself as
"Sore Throat"—a takeoff on Deep Throat of the Watergate
scandal—sent copies of anti-chiropractic articles that had
appeared in newspapers across the country to the NCAC.
"Dr. Throat" only identified himself as a medical doctor
who was bothered by what he had seen in the internal
files at the AMA and offered to do what he could to help
rectify the unjust things he had seen happening.[59]

George McAndrews, an experienced antitrust lawyer
from Chicago, accepted the case on behalf of chiropractors
and cited his reason for doing so was that his father had
been dying from a severe case of asthma in 1928 when

after only three visits to a chiropractor, his asthma went away, and he never had another attack. His father was so impressed with the healing he'd experienced under chiropractic care that he became a chiropractor himself. McAndrews remembered his father's frustration that his beloved profession was either ignored or denigrated, often by the very people who could have benefited from chiropractic.

The court case was a true David and Goliath scenario. The AMA seemed to have unlimited funds with which to fight for their interests. Chiropractors across the country supported the effort as best as they could. In the four years it took to get to court, McAndrews traveled to 34 states and took depositions from 165 witnesses. Over one million documents were collected, some that boldly stated the AMA's intent to contain and eliminate chiropractic. Documents contained statements like the following: "If this program is successfully pursued, it is entirely likely that chiropractic as a profession will wither and die on the vine, and the chiropractic menace will die a natural but somewhat un-dramatic death." A recorded statement from a Joseph Sabatier, MD, at an AMA Committee on Quackery meeting said that "Alerting young physicians to the dangers of chiropractic has been neglected, and that [he, the young MD, has] the problem of starting a practice, and it would be well to get across the point that the chiropractor is stealing [his] money."[5] Document by document, McAndrews painted a picture of the AMA's broad-based conspiracy to destroy the chiropractic profession.

Every MD who took the stand was given the opportunity to give some example demonstrating that chiropractic does not work, and none could. H. Doyl Taylor, an attorney and the director of the AMA's Department of Investigation, and the secretary of the AMA Committee on Quackery, conveniently moved out of Chicago the Friday before the trial started, leaving the jurisdiction of the court. His son testified that Mr. Taylor had crippling arthritis and was unable to return to Chicago. (However, a private investigator discovered that Mr. Taylor was healthy enough to play golf nearly every day in Arizona.)

The presiding judge, Judge Nicholas Bua, had little experience in antitrust suits, which troubled the plaintiffs. After a seven-week trial, the jury returned a verdict of not guilty within two hours.

Disappointment turned to anger, and in January 1982, before a three-judge panel, McAndrews presented 13 errors that had been made in the trial, which included improper jury instructions and the admission of irrelevant and prejudicial evidence. On September 19, 1983, the U.S. Court of Appeals unanimously agreed and ordered a new trial.

Chester A. Wilk and the three other chiropractors named as plaintiffs in the suit decided to forego a jury trial (and a right to sue for damages). This would keep the focus on antitrust where it belonged and show that the chiropractors were interested in principle, not money.

On May 5, 1987, *Wilk v. AMA* was back in court, this time to seek only injunctive relief, a court order to prevent the medical establishment from continuing its boycott of chiropractic. The presiding judge, Judge Susan Getzendanner, had a reputation for being no-nonsense, knowledgeable, efficient, and fast.

This time McAndrews brought in some of the finest medical doctors in the country to testify as expert witnesses on the behalf of chiropractors, something he had not done in the previous trial. Among them was Dr. John Mennell, a world-renowned orthopedist who had been a professor at eight different medical schools and written several textbooks and many articles in medical journals. Dr. Mennell testified that "if you ask new residents how long they spent studying problems of the musculoskeletal system, they would reply, 'zero to about four hours.'" When the AMA's lawyers asked Dr. Mennell if, since the musculoskeletal system accounts for 60% of the body, was he saying the entire medical school curriculum is devoted to about 40% of the body, Dr. Mennell replied, "Yes, sir."

This time, studies were presented to the court as evidence that chiropractic care worked. Among them were two independent studies that showed chiropractic care was able to get people back to work in half the time and at half the cost of medical care. One of these was a report by Rolland A. Martin, MD, Medical Director for the Oregon Workmen's Compensation Board.

"Relief here is provided not only to the plaintiff chiropractors, but also in a sense to all consumers of health care services."

U.S. Court of Appeals,
Wilk v. American Medical Association,
February 7, 1990

D. Per Freitag, another medical doctor, testified that patients in one hospital who received chiropractic treatment were released sooner than patients in another hospital that did not allow chiropractors.

H. Doyl Taylor, who was too sick to come back to Chicago and testify about his work with the AMA at the last trial, was, once again, summoned for this trial, and, once again, Taylor insisted he was not well enough to make the trip. McAndrews got permission to go to Arizona and get his testimony on videotape. When Taylor insisted he was too ill to testify on video, Judge Getzendanner issued a court order mandating that the AMA have Taylor submit to a physical exam. Thinking that an exam by an MD or chiropractor might introduce bias, Taylor was examined by an osteopath, who pronounced him in excellent health. During the questioning, Taylor made a startling admission: He said that when he took the position with the AMA as director of the Department of Investigation and acting secretary of AMA's Committee on Quackery, he did not know "a chiropractor from an antelope and still had only a vague idea of what chiropractors did."[60]

Another crucial document surfaced during the second trial—a letter that had been sent by Irvin Hendryson, MD, an orthopedic surgeon and an AMA trustee, to Robert Throckmorton, the AMA's general counsel. In the letter, Dr. Hendryson reported on a controlled study of orthopedic versus chiropractic care that had been conducted in a military orthopedic ward during WWII. The study showed that chiropractic had impressive successes with some cases in which medical treatment had failed, concluding that chiropractic adjustments were at least as effective as some of the best medical treatments. Dr. Hendryson suggested that chiropractic be made available in all hospital ortho-pedic wards. The contents of this letter proved beyond doubt that the AMA and its Committee on Quackery had known all along that chiropractic was effective.

On August 27, 1987, Judge Susan Getzendanner handed down her 101-page decision finding the American Medical Association, the American College of Radiology, the American College of Surgeons, and the American Academy of Orthopaedic Surgeons *guilty,* as alleged, of joining a conspiracy against chiropractors in violation of antitrust law. One month later, Judge Getzendanner issued an in-junction forbidding the AMA to engage in any collective boycott against chiropractors and forcing the AMA to tell its members that the organization's official position *now* was that it *was* ethical for medical doctors to associate professionally with chiropractors. The AMA was directed to send a copy of this order to each AMA member and employee, first class, postage prepaid, within 30 days of the entry of the order or to send mailing labels to the court clerk and let the court mail out notices of the order.

The judge also ordered the AMA to publish the court order in the *Journal of the American Medical Association* (JAMA), indexed under "Chiropractic" so it could be easily found. Lastly, the AMA had to file a report with the court by January 10, 1988, showing that it had complied with the judge's order.

Of course, the AMA appealed Judge Getzendanner's decision, but less than three years later, on February 7, 1990, the United States Court of Appeals found that the conspiracy against chiropractic did indeed constitute an antitrust injury, rather than a free speech issue, as the AMA claimed. The opinion from the appellate court included this statement:

> Relief here is provided not only to the plaintiff chiropractors, but also in a sense to all consumers of health care services. Ensuring that medical physicians and hospitals are free to professionally associate with chiropractors likely will eliminate such anticompetitive effects of the boycott as interfering with consumers' free choice in choosing product (health care providers) of their liking.[61]

The AMA took their appeal to the U.S. Supreme Court three times, but the Supreme Court declined to hear the case. Following a decade of litigation, the Seventh Circuit Court upheld the ruling by U.S. District Court Judge Getzendanner that the AMA had engaged in a "lengthy, systematic, accessible and unlawful boycott" designed to restrict operation between MDs and chiropractors in order to eliminate the profession of chiropractic.[62]

Except for the attorneys who represented chiropractors, no one received one penny from the settlement, an effort that was supported financially by chiropractors all across the country giving what they could to fight for their profession.

In an ideal world, chiropractors, after winning a 16-year-long legal battle against a powerhouse like the AMA, would have the integrity of their profession restored and they could, with dignity and pride, from that point on, take their rightful place among health care providers. But just as many segments of the American population who have fought for their rights under the law and "won" will tell you just because you had your day in court doesn't mean the prejudice goes away. Sometimes it's still pervasive, just more subtle. My guess is that some who are reading this right now have a bias against chiropractic that they would be hard-pressed to explain.

Over 40 years ago, a popular ad asked, "How do you spell relief?" It was reported that across the nation when school children were asked to actually spell the word *relief,* they answered, "R-o-l-a-i-d-s," just like some of you just did. When we hear something over and over, or even occasionally—sometimes just once from someone whose opinion we value—we tend to remember it and more importantly, believe it, often without ever questioning whether or not it's true or accurate. Joseph E. Levine, an Oscar-winning movie promoter, said, "You can fool all the people all the time if the advertising is right and the budget is big enough."

Likewise, what we read can have a powerful impact on what we accept as true, especially if it comes from what we consider a reliable source. Even if it's later proven *untrue,* the story that sticks in our mind is the one that made the headlines, not the retraction that appeared days or weeks later buried somewhere on the back page. Too often, innocent people targeted by false accusations continue to suffer from the bad publicity.

Prejudice simply means to pre-judge, to form an opinion without the facts or experience to back it up. I think most of the prejudice chiropractors still have to deal with stems from the bad press the profession endured at the hands of the American Medical Association years ago, even though it was proven wrong in a court of law. I've had people tell me that they "don't believe in chiropractors," to which I usually respond, "Really? Touch me. I'm real." Almost always, after talking to these folks awhile, I realize they have *no idea* how I work with patients; many believe chiropractors just "crack backs," and some have never even been to a chiropractor of any kind! If that's not pre-judging, what is? Occasionally, someone will tell me he went to a chiropractor once, that the adjustment hurt—Upper Cervical adjustments do *not* hurt—and it didn't help, so "chiropractic doesn't work." Judging a whole group by a limited experience is also a definition of prejudice. That's like saying because the food at one restaurant wasn't good, I'm going to stop eating out. For that matter, I bet most people have gone to MDs or taken drugs that didn't seem to help them, but that didn't stop them from going to another doctor or taking another pill.

But the good news is—and I tell patients this—people get better regardless of what they believe. Just like they don't have to believe in gravity for it to work, they don't have to believe in Upper Cervical Care for it to work.

I could fill this book writing about the people and businesses hurt by slanderous reports that were later proved to be untrue. In 1994, it was reported that the president of Proctor & Gamble appeared on *The Phil Donahue Show* and announced that he was a Satanist and that a large portion of P&G's profits went to support the Church of Satan. Incredibly, a lot of people believed that story! It was soon proven that P&G's president was never on *Donahue*, and how the company directs its profits is a matter of public record. But the truth didn't stop the attacks from

mounting, and in 1998, it was reported that the CEO of
P&G made the same admission about the company donat-
ing part of its profits to the Church of Satan, this time on
The Sally Jesse Raphael Show. Again, it was proven that
no one representing Proctor & Gamble had ever appeared
on *The Sally Jesse Raphael Show*. Although it was never
determined who started the rumor, in March 2007, a jury
awarded P&G $19.25 million after finding that four Amway
distributors had spread the false rumor about P&G to
advance their own businesses.[63]

At the end of World War II, a group of German prison-
ers of war, high-ranking officers of the Third Reich, were
being brought to the United States. During the war these
Germans had read articles and been shown pictures of the
"bombing of New York Harbor," all fabricated and circulated by the Nazi's Minister of Propaganda. The Germans
laughed at the Americans who told them New York had
never been bombed during the war. When they pulled
into the harbor and saw for themselves that New York
was still standing, the Germans marveled that America
could rebuild such a large city so fast.[64]

What's my point? We are all influenced by what we
read and what we hear over and over. It has nothing to
do with intelligence; it's just how our minds work. And I
really believe many people have a prejudice against chiropractic that stems not from their knowledge or personal
experience with the profession, but from the bad press
chiropractors suffered at the hands of the AMA when they,
as U.S. District Court Judge Getzendanner's decision,
stated "engaged in a lengthy, systematic, accessible and
unlawful boycott designed to restrict operation between

MDs and chiropractors in order to *eliminate* the profession of chiropractic."

Yes, the case was settled in favor of chiropractic in 1987, but the prejudice against chiropractic didn't disappear with the ruling that found chiropractors not guilty of the accusations the American Medical Association made against them. Prejudice is taught, and we can carry it for generations, sometimes on a subconscious level.

How many medical doctors, knowingly or unknowingly, pass their own negative views of chiropractic to others—their families, their co-workers, their friends, their patients? Ask any chiropractor and he/she will tell you that some medical doctors are still telling their patients that chiropractic is quackery, a bogus practice that won't help them. We know they are because when their patients finally do come to us, *they tell us!* Why are so many in the medical profession still denigrating or denying the value of chiropractic, especially after the mounting scientific evidence of the last 117 years that proves its efficacy in treating so much disease?

How do you spell relief?

The fact that the AMA called chiropractors *quacks* used to really ruffle my feathers. Then I realized maybe being called a quack wasn't so bad.

Galileo, the Italian astronomer now called the "Father of Modern Science," was called a quack by his detractors. He was thrown in prison for heresy and tortured until he renounced his scientific beliefs.

Thomas Edison was called a quack. It took him 15 years, from 1870-1885, to overcome the prejudice of his countrymen and get them to install electric lights.

William Röntgen, German scientist and inventor of X-rays, was another "quack," much criticized in the papers because it was said he would invade the privacy of the boudoir with invisible rays.

Samuel F. B. Morse, inventor of the telegraph, was also called a quack. His first appeal to Congress for aid in developing the telegraph was flatly refused, and Morse spent his entire fortune before his invention was approved.

Charles Goodyear, who gave the world vulcanized rubber, was another famous "quack." The public called him a fool and an imbecile. He almost starved before he was successful.

The baby buggy was invented by a "quack" named Charles Burton. His invention was outlawed as a traffic menace.

In 1865, a Boston newspaper reported that Joshua Coppersmith, 46, was arrested trying to peddle telephone stock, although the paper said Mr. Coppersmith was "attempting to extort funds from ignorant and superstitious people by exhibiting a device which he said would convey the human voice over any distance through metallic wires so that it would be heard by the listener at the other end. Only a 'quack' would try such a thing."[65]

On the other hand, American newspapers refused to publish the news that on December 17, 1903, Wilbur and Orville Wright had flown a heavier-than-air machine. The brothers offered the United States War Department all rights to the invention, but Uncle Sam's boys were too shrewd to be taken in. Leading scientists had explained that flying machines were impossible, and the Wright brothers' letters went into the "crank file."[66]

Being called a quack turned out all right for those guys. Maybe I should lighten up on the subject.

I'm not trying to insult anybody; I'm just trying to debunk some of the myths about chiropractic in general and educate folks about Upper Cervical in particular. Socrates said, "The unexamined life is not worth living," and I'm just saying that unexamined beliefs can make life a lot harder (and more painful), too.

"It is harder to crack a prejudice than an atom."

Albert Einstein

In the documentary *The Power of Upper Cervical,* a colleague shares a story about a patient who came to him who had been diagnosed with Ménière's disease and was suffering terribly. Her world would just spin, as she described it, without warning. Her former husband was a medical doctor at the most prominent medical university in the state and had seen to it that she got the best medical treatment the center had to offer. She was on a salt-free diet and several medications; they had tried everything.

After she got under Upper Cervical Care, the Ménière's went away. She had five children, and she got them all under Upper Cervical Care, as well. She had a daughter who was suffering from headaches and was having menstrual cycles only every three to four months. After a while, the daughter's menstrual cycle normalized and the headaches went away. Another child had insomnia and would fall asleep in school. After Upper Cervical corrections, his insomnia cleared up.

"To hold to one assumption and deny all contradictory data is not science—that is politics."

Anonymous

One day the woman's former husband, the medical doctor, called the Upper Cervical doctor and told him he had allergic rhinitis, which has allergy-type symptoms, and that he wanted to get under Upper Cervical Care. About two to three weeks into care, the medical doctor had seen some improvement in his rhinitis, but said to the Upper Cervical doctor, "I have to tell you something. Something has happened to me, and I can't explain it. Before I started care with you, I had a severe case of impotency for years, and it's completely, 100% cleared up. What did you do?"

About three months later, the woman asked the Upper Cervical doctor if her physician ex-husband had referred any cases to him because she said he talked about cases that he thought medical care was not helping. The Upper Cervical doctor answered, "Not one."

This man's father was also a medical doctor, a highly respected internist who was still practicing. The woman told the Upper Cervical doctor later that when she asked her former husband why he had not referred any cases to Upper Cervical Care, he had said, "What would my colleagues and my father think if I referred patients to a chiropractor?"

This kind of thing happens to chiropractors all the time, to the detriment of those who might be helped by chiropractic care.

Another perception some people have of chiropractors is that we're not as educated as medical doctors. I think some people even think we chiropractors aren't very smart—if we were, we would've gone to medical school and become a "real" doctor. What these people don't understand is that there are ways of healing other than drugs and surgery, and some practitioners in the healing arts prefer those other ways, chiropractors among them. If you're thinking that this is another prejudice against chiropractors that sticks in my craw, you would be correct.

In fact, that was part of the AMA's defense in the 1980 lawsuit: that chiropractors' education was inferior to that of medical doctors. In response to this, McAndrews, attorney for the chiropractors, proposed to the judge that the entire jury be taken to the National College of Chiropractic in Lombard, Illinois, less than an hour away, so they could see firsthand what a chiropractic education consists of and assess the quality of the teaching. However, the defense attorneys had been taken on a tour of National before the case went to trial, and they had seen what the college had to offer. Attorneys for the AMA fought against McAndrews's proposal, so the jury never had the opportunity to witness what chiropractic education truly is.[67]

Chiropractic colleges are accredited by the Council on Chiropractic Education, a federally approved accrediting organization operating under the U.S. Department of Education, in much the same way medical schools are. Before chiropractors can practice, they must be licensed by their state. All states require them to pass four National Chiropractic Board examinations.

A study comparing chiropractic to medical school education found that on average, chiropractic school education required 4,800 hours to complete and medical school required 4,667 hours. The studied chiropractic schools taught an average of 290 more hours in the basic sciences than did the medical counterparts. However, medical school focuses a higher portion of its program on clinical sciences and internships, with chiropractic training being more didactic. As was noted by the medical doctor who was called as a witness in *Wilk v. AMA*, this study also found that chiropractors receive much more education on the musculoskeletal system than medical doctors.[68]

A study of 85 recent medical school graduates taking a 25-question test that had been validated by 124 orthopedic chairpersons for basic competency in musculoskeletal medicine found that the mean score for all residents in their first postgraduate year was 59.6%. Seventy of the 85, or 82%, failed to demonstrate basic competency. This is a concern because musculoskeletal symptoms rank second only to respiratory illness as the most common reason patients seek medical attention.[69]

Finally, the following table appeared in September 2010 on the RAND Corporation's website, in an article titled "Changing Views of Chiropractic: A Comparison of Chiropractic and Medical School Curriculum." (The RAND Corporation—RAND stands for research and development—is an independent, highly respected, nonprofit global think tank.)

Characteristics	Chiropractic Schools		Medical Schools	
	Average Hours (all US schools)	% of total contact hours	Avg. Hours (all U.S. schools)	% of total contact hours
Total contact	4,826	100	4,867	100
Basic sciences	1,420	29	1,200	26
Clinical experiences prior to graduation	1,406	29	3,487	74
Clinical sciences	3,406	71	3,487	70
Chiropractic sciences	1,975	41	NA	NA

www.rand.org/pubs/research_briefs

This is not to suggest that the field of medicine is peopled with less than highly intelligent, highly educated, and highly skilled professionals. It is. *My* only intent is to correct the misperceptions that many people still have about chiropractic.

"It's better to light one candle than to curse the darkness."

B. J. Palmer

✳ ✳ ✳

Sandy H., Upper Cervical Patient
Suffered from back pain and injuries related to a car accident

I was involved in a head-on collision over 20 years ago. A teenage driver crossed the center line and hit my car, which went down an embankment. I felt okay right after the accident, but a few days later, the pain hit me.

I remember it well because I was Christmas shopping at the time. I had mostly muscle damage, so I went to a general chiropractor for my injuries. I had lower back pain for 10 years following the accident; the pain was always there. Every time I brushed my teeth, vacuumed, did laundry, or anything, my back hurt, but I just tried to deal with it and live my life.

Then, about 10 years ago, I got sick, and nobody could tell me what was wrong with me. I was so tired I didn't want to get out of bed. My hands and legs tingled. I could hardly eat. My husband gave me Ensure, so I'd get some nutrition. For four to five months I couldn't eat solid food. I lost 60 pounds.

So I started going to doctors, trying to find out what was wrong with me. I had a spinal tap, which came back fine. Then I had an MRI, which showed that I had more lesions on my brain than I was supposed to have at my age. So based on the lesions, I was diagnosed with multiple sclerosis, and they wanted to put me on medication for MS. I said no, not yet, because I don't do a lot of drugs.

I did some research on lesions and found that rheumatic fever and scarlet fever could also cause lesions on the brain. Well, I'd had scarlet fever twice in my life. So that, and not multiple sclerosis, could be the reason I had more lesions. I just never believed that I had MS, and I think you have to listen to your own body.

One day shortly after this, I was in the dentist office with my kids, and I saw an ad in Charlotte Woman *for Upper Cervical Care that said, "Have You Been Diagnosed with Multiple Sclerosis?" Well, that got my attention. So I took the magazine home with me. Yes,*

I stole it, so I'd have this ad about Upper Cervical to show my husband.

The next day, my husband and I were at a home improvement show uptown, and lo and behold, Upper Cervical had a display there. So, I say to myself, okay, this is a God thing. I have got to stop and talk to these people. That's how I found out about Upper Cervical Care.

Now the healing was slow for me, but I felt better every time I went for an Upper Cervical adjustment. It took a couple of years to get 99% of my health back. I tell everybody I see who's starting Upper Cervical Care to have patience. You have to be in it for the long haul if you want to see a difference. I know some people get better right away, but it took my body awhile; but you have to remember, I had that car accident over 20 years ago. I'm almost positive that accident was the cause of everything my body's been through since.

It took a couple of years to get my body back, but like I said, I kept feeling better and better with each adjustment. And there came a time when, I don't know, maybe I had been under Upper Cervical Care for a year or so, when Doug, my husband, and I were having trouble with a well, and we had to pull a pump out of this well. I remember being bent over, pulling the pump out of the well, when I was hit with the awareness that I didn't have any pain in my back. And I haven't had any pain in my back since. None.

For years I'd had this pain in the background. I'd tell myself that I wasn't going to think about it, but it was still there, all the time. That day, pulling the pump out of the well, I actually had the thought that my back should really be hurting now, when I realized I had no pain whatsoever. I'm absolutely fine now. I just go to my Upper Cervical doctor for maintenance every two weeks, because my body was so whacked, it won't hold the adjustment longer than two weeks. Plus, I'm under a lot of stress—when you're in business for yourself, it can be stressful—so I go to Upper Cervical Care to boost my immune system because of the stress, as well. I've gotten to the point where I pretty much know when I need an adjustment. Now my husband, Doug, will hold an adjustment longer. He goes for maintenance once a month. He's my second story.

Doug was thrown from a lawn mower and broke his back. Upper Cervical helped him heal, so he didn't have to have surgery. Doug went to Upper Cervical because of me. He'd seen how my body came back under Upper Cervical Care, so he believed he could get better without surgery, and he did. He had a lot of joint pain in his legs and knees; he doesn't have that anymore.

My sister also went to Upper Cervical. She had irritable bowel syndrome and really bad headaches. Plus, she was on a lot of antidepressants. She had so much going on with her body. She started seeing a difference under Upper Cervical Care, then she stopped going. She said she couldn't afford it. I said, "What do you mean you can't afford it? Did you consider how often you miss work? Look at the drugs you're taking that cost you." She takes pain pills, sleeping pills, and antidepressants. So she's back to her same ol', same ol', and she complains all the time about how bad she feels.

I feel like saying, I don't want to hear it. You found the help you needed. You were getting better, and you quit it, so that's the consequence. I can't feel sorry for anybody when they make those kinds of choices. It's like some people would rather have surgery than try a drug-free, natural approach to healing like Upper Cervical Care that really works.

I've sent a lot of people to Upper Cervical Care, but sometimes I hesitate. Like a couple of days ago, someone on Facebook was asking for a recommendation for a doctor to work with a child who had ADHD, and I almost told her about Upper Cervical, but I didn't, because I knew I'd get flack from a lot of people online, and I just didn't want to deal with all that. But I wish they could've seen some of the patients I've seen in the 10 years I've been going to Upper Cervical. I remember this one little boy who was one of those amazing miracles; that's all you can say. When I first saw him, he couldn't talk. He just made animal-like sounds. Autism. I saw the transformation in this little boy, over time, and we went to a dinner one night and they were there, and the little boy talked. He talked!

Even my 88-year-old dad, who comes down from Michigan during the winter, got under Upper Cervical Care while he was here, and we saw such an amazing change in him. My dad has diabetes and has to give himself shots, the whole nine yards. He had these places on his hand; he couldn't feel his fingers. Plus, my dad was all bent over; he's this little old man. Dad grew at least two inches after his first adjustment. He was standing straight and tall with his shoulders pulled back. I was so proud of him. At the end of the four to six weeks that Dad went to my Upper Cervical doctor, he could feel his fingers. Now the sad thing is, there are no Upper Cervical doctors where he lives, so when I saw him in July, Dad's body was all hunched over again and he couldn't feel his fingers.

When you see people like Doug and me, at age 50 and over, having been through what we've been through, feeling good and on no drugs whatsoever, something's working, and it's Upper Cervical Care. Doug and I don't have health insurance; Upper Cervical Care is our health insurance, and it has been for the last 10 years. I consider my Upper Cervical doctor to be my primary care doctor.

I have had people tell me stuff like all chiropractors are quacks, that what we experienced with Upper Cervical is all in our head. I tell them, "You know what? If it's all in my head, so be it, because it works." They can say what they want to about it. All I know is doctors told me I had MS, and I didn't, or if I did, I don't anymore. I feel really good now, and it's all because of Upper Cervical Care.

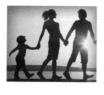

CHAPTER 9

The Research

"If it is a miracle, any sort of evidence will answer, but if it is a fact, proof is necessary."

Mark Twain

The fact is, very little in the health care profession has been proven beyond a shadow of a doubt. Research is not a project but a process. In looking at data to support a particular intervention, one must consider efficacy, reliability, safety, and cost-effectiveness. The purpose of this book is to provide evidence that Upper Cervical Health Care is an excellent health care system by all four measures.

It will come as no surprise to learn that you will not find as many research studies in Upper Cervical Care as you will find studies on drugs or medical procedures. The reason for this is simple: A natural healing procedure has no product to patent and potentially profit from; therefore, chiropractic does not have the deep pockets of the pharmaceutical industry or any other for-profit entity to support its research. Most of the studies you're about to read were performed by Upper Cervical doctors and sometimes medical doctors who saw the need to validate the success patients were getting under Upper Cervical Care.

A word about research methods: The randomized controlled trial (RCT) is considered the gold standard in research design, but it does not typically represent what takes place in practice. Therefore, practice-based research (PBR) is a valuable alternative to the randomized controlled trial. Practice-based research attempts to answer the bottom-line question, "Is the care effective?"[70] Isn't that the question anyone suffering from anything wants answered?

A paper published by the Department of Internal Medicine and Yale University School of Medicine titled "Randomized, Controlled Trials and Observational Studies and the Hierarchy of Research Design" concluded well-designed observational studies do not systematically overestimate the magnitude of the effects of treatment as compared with those in randomized controlled trials of the same topic. The study shows that the case-control report may have more scientific merit than it has been given credit for in the past.[71]

However, in this chapter, I present evidence from both research methods that shows the effectiveness of Upper Cervical Care. For readers who would like to dive more deeply into the research that has been done in Upper Cervical since B. J. Palmer, I would direct them to Dr. Kirk Eriksen's brilliant book, *Upper Cervical Subluxation Complex: A Review of the Chiropractic and Medical Literature*. Although it is written more for the practitioner than the layperson, it is worth the effort, and the Editorial Comments at the end of each section contain helpful summaries. Dr. Eriksen's book contains hundreds of papers and studies that support the effectiveness of Upper Cervical Care. One chapter alone contains over 90 published Upper Cervical case studies, over 50% of those from peer-reviewed journals.

The following is a sample of Upper Cervical research studies listed in alphabetical order by ailment:

Athletic Injuries: Four different studies—one on basketball players, one on football players, one on baseball players, and one on cyclers—establish the relationship between body structure or biomechanics to both athletic injuries and success in that sport. The evidence appears to show that doctors of chiropractic are the leading specialists in spinal structural correction, so it makes sense that this is the type of doctor who should play a major role in the care of athletes. Chiropractic care has been shown to enhance the performance of world-class athletes and regular fitness enthusiasts alike. One other benefit that is just as important is that people who are under regular chiropractic care have a reduced risk of injury. Who knows how many injuries have *not* had to be rehabilitated because they had been *prevented* by regular chiropractic care.[72]

A research study conducted by Drs. Anthony Lauro and Brian Mouch, published in the *Journal of Chiropractic Research and Clinical Investigation*, indicated chiropractic care might improve athletic performance by as much as 16.7% over a two-week period. The report also concluded that subluxation-free athletes react faster, coordinate better, and execute finer movements with improved accuracy and precision, resulting in an overall better athlete.

Auditory Dysfunctions: AGJ Terrett did a comprehensive review of studies showing an association between cervical dysfunction and hearing deficit with cervical adjustments improving audio metric function.[73] (Remember, the very first chiropractic patient had his hearing restored by an upper cervical adjustment.)

Blood Pressure Study: A 2007 study conducted by two medical doctors, Dr. George Bakris, Director of the Hypertension Center at the University of Chicago Medical Center, and Dr. Bruce Bell, a family practitioner, showed that a one-time Upper Cervical adjustment of a misaligned C1 (atlas) vertebra significantly reduced blood pressure in people with hypertension (high blood pressure). Fifty patients with high blood pressure were sent to Dr. Marshall Dickholtz, Sr., an Upper Cervical doctor in Chicago. Twenty-five received an Upper Cervical adjustment; the other 25 received a sham intervention. Patients were assessed after the alignment and again after eight weeks. [74]

"We were shocked to find out that we got more than double what we expected in blood pressure reduction in the patients who received the Upper Cervical adjustment. These patients did not need to resume taking blood pressure medicine and the effect lasted for months. This procedure (an Upper Cervical adjustment) has the effect of not one, but two blood-pressure medications given in combination, and it seems to be adverse-event free. We saw no side effects and no problems," Dr. Bakris told the *Chicago Tribune* and WebMD.[75]

Carpal Tunnel Syndrome (CTS): Stress to the median nerve commonly begins in the neck. The nerve is then aggravated by added pressure or irritation anywhere from the neck to the wrist, which can then cause symptoms in the hands and fingers. This is called "double crush syndrome" and is widely referenced in the scientific and medical research journals as a consistent finding in patients with carpal tunnel syndrome. Pressure or irritation to the nerve roots as they exit the neck makes the median nerve more vulnerable to injury at the wrist.

The medical journal *The Lancet* found that seven out of every 10 CTS patients had nerve irritation in the neck, which suggests the majority of CTS patients actually have double crush phenomena.[76] This would explain the high failure rate of common medical treatments—braces, splints, over-the-counter or prescription non-steroidal anti-inflammatory drugs (NSAIDs), cortisone injections, or surgery—and points to the need to first correct the cervical problem (by an Upper Cervical correction) to allow the wrist condition to fully heal.

Diabetes: Research conducted at the Hospital for Sick Children and the University of Calgary discovered there is a "control circuit" necessary to retain the health and normal function of the cells that produce insulin located in the pancreas between insulin-producing cells and nerves. (This "control circuit" has long been known within the Upper Cervical profession as the "brain-to-body communication circuit.") As part of the study, scientists "knocked out" specific nerve cells and discovered that doing so created an interference with the brain-to-body communication.

These nerve cells had a direct and profound effect on the pancreas, diabetes, and blood sugar levels and the research concluded that the nerves are critical in the development of diabetes.[77]

This helps explain a condition that diabetics often suffer from called peripheral neuropathy, a numbness or pain described as a burning sensation or a feeling like pins and needles being stuck in the arms or legs. The research suggests that neuropathy may be more than a result of diabetes; it may be related to the nervous system's role in the whole disease process.

Disease (in general): Dr. Tsun-Nin Lee from the Academy of Pain Research in San Francisco, in a paper titled "Thalamic Neuron Theory: Theoretical Basis for the Role Played by the Central Nervous System in the Causes and Cures of All Diseases," suggests something chiropractors have known for more than 100 years: that the central nervous system controls and regulates virtually every function in the body, and thus dysfunction to the neuroaxis plays a role in many disease processes.[78]

Fibromyalgia: Although the cause of fibromyalgia is not fully understood, studies and clinical trials show that fibromyalgia can develop after traumatic neck injuries. Renowned neurosurgeon Dr. Michael Rosner states that when the neck is hyper-extended, the spinal canal narrows, impacting the spine and the brain stem. This can occur in cases of whiplash in automobile accidents, extended dental work in which the head is bent back, or severe bouts of coughing. Even activities like painting a ceiling can cause injury to the neck that can lead to fibromyalgia.[79]

Headaches: It has been estimated that each year, 45 million Americans get chronic, recurring headaches. One in four households has a migraine sufferer, and migraine sufferers lose more than 157,000,000 workdays each year, costing business and industry more than 50 billion dollars in lost productivity and medical expenses. More than four billion dollars are spent annually on over-the-counter pain relievers for headaches.[80]

In one study, relationships with family and friends were negatively impacted for 89% of the respondents who suffered from headaches. The medical management of these headaches consists of various medications and, in certain cases, trigger-point injections. The medical approach is usually directed toward treatment of symptoms as opposed to a possible cause. Chiropractors have been helping patients with headaches for more than 100 years. Research suggests that adverse tension from cervical joint dysfunctions could cause cervicogenic headaches.[81]

In an article in the *Journal of the American Medical Association* (JAMA), E. Seletz discusses how most headaches related to whiplash are from an injury to the C2 nerve root. He points out that the vulnerability of the nerve root is due to the fact that there are no pedicles or facet joints in the upper cervical region. He states that many "headaches are not headaches at all, but really a pain in the neck." Seletz also discusses the vulnerability of the vertebral artery and upper cervical spine and how this can be injured in a whiplash. He relates the following symptoms to disturbed blood flow in the vertebral artery: vertigo, migraine-like headaches, nausea and vomiting, disturbed speech and swallowing, and unsteadiness of gait.[82]

The Department of Anesthesiology at the UCLA School of Medicine tried to determine whether the pain from cervicogenic headaches could be due to referred symptoms from myofascial trigger points. Of the 11 patients studied, 10 had specific segmental dysfunction of the upper spine. The author concluded that cervical segmental dysfunction is a common finding with these patients and recommended that conservative care be provided before surgery.[83]

Another study examined a group of 12 children complaining of severe headaches. The study group was compared to a matched group of 12 headache-free children. The results showed the children suffering from severe headaches had very tense neck muscles.[84]

A study out of Norway made the following statement in reference to the importance of the cervical spine: "Not only a passive role—that of a link between the head and the rest of the body—is allotted to the neck. All its important structures make it a critical part of the body. With his own local motion, man can make up to around 40 km/h. The dimensions and the structure of the neck have not been designed for modern velocities and their inherent accidents."[85]

In a controlled clinical trial, Drs. Boline, Kassak, Nelson, and Anderson studied spinal manipulation versus amitriptyline for the treatment of chronic, tension-type headaches. The data reveal not only that chiropractic adjustments are safer than drug therapy, but they also provide longer-lasting relief than amitriptyline medication. Another study of 5,520 patients suffering from headaches stated that drug-induced headaches occur frequently.[86]

These studies from both the medical and chiropractic literature show a correlation between cervical biomechanical dysfunction and headaches.

Immune System Disorders: Dr. D.R. Murray from the Department of Medicine at the University of California discussed the growing evidence suggesting that the immune function is regulated in part by the sympathetic nervous system, and the sympathetic nervous system has the highest amount of regulatory input coming from the atlas region. Another paper published by D.L. Felton discussed the direct neural connection of the central nervous system to the immune system.[87]

A review paper from a team of doctors at the National Institute of Health discussed how the brain and immune system talk to each other and how this process is essential to maintaining homeostasis.[88] If the subluxation influences the central nervous system with concomitant immune system dysfunction, then its removal may give the patient's innate healing ability an improved chance of dealing with his health condition.

Multiple Sclerosis: Dr. Charles Poser of the Harvard Medical School concluded in his published article, "Trauma to the Central Nervous System May Result in Formation or Enlargement of Multiple Sclerosis Plaques," that trauma to the head, neck, or upper back can act as a trigger for the appearance of new or recurrent symptoms in some patients with MS. He stated further that only trauma affecting the brain and/or spinal cord can be considered significant.[89] Dr. Poser suggested there is a relationship between trauma and the aggravation or creation of multiple sclerosis. (However, MS may not develop for months or even years after the injury.)

Upper Cervical chiropractors have always had evidence from PBR, practice-based research; we see patients getting well every day, but now we've also begun to get validation that Upper Cervical Care works from RCT, randomized controlled trials, and that's exciting. Now, I'd like to mix it up a bit and have Dr. Mandolesi and Dr. Marceca share, via narrative, the research Dr. Mandolesi is currently conducting in Italy with MS patients under Upper Cervical Care. This is how they relayed their story to my assistant:

"I first heard about Upper Cervical Care from Damiana's husband, who is a friend of mine," Dr. Marceca said. "I was really surprised when I saw how much Damiana had improved after getting Upper Cervical Care in America. It was difficult for me to believe that chiropractic care could help a chronic, degenerative disease like Damiana had, but I couldn't deny the improvement I saw with my own eyes in her mobility." (Damiana's story is at the end of Chapter Six.)

"I am a curious person, and I think, an open-minded one," Dr. Marceca continued, "so I went to the Internet to research Upper Cervical Health Centers and this Dr. Drury. In June of 2008, I met Dr. Drury in Italy and asked to speak with some of his patients, which I did, both in Italy and later in the United States. Patients in both places told me they were getting well from all sorts of conditions, and I could see Dr. Drury's belief in and passion for the Upper Cervical work.

"Something else happened for me to know there was something here I had to explore. In 2008, in San Marino,

I saw a patient there, Maurizio Garuffi, who had been under Upper Cervical Care for eight, nine months. He was maybe 35 years old, and he said before Upper Cervical Care, he could not move his arms. He moved his arms for me, and I was so impressed by this I promised him I would come back and see him in six months, which I did in May 2009. Now, this man told me he had not been under any other care, only Upper Cervical, and that he was not taking medications—this is important to know. This second time I saw Maurizio, he could stand alone, something he couldn't do before. He was even able to walk with assistance. I get emotional telling the story. We are men of science, no? But when you see this, you realize all the possibilities to help our patients."

"The problem, as I see it, between medical doctors and chiropractors, is lack of understanding."

Dr. Sandro Mandolesi, MD

"So I contacted my friend from Sardinia, Dr. Mandolesi, this marvelous brain who works with MS patients and shared with him all this. He, too, gets very interested. We talk with Dr. Drury and, before long, start doing research with, in the beginning, just eight MS patients from all over Italy who were under care at one of Dr. Drury's Upper Cervical clinics. Now, we have formed a collaboration with other medical doctors here in Italy who are also interested in our findings. We all realize this is very important research."

"The preliminary results of our research on how Upper Cervical Care can help patients with multiple sclerosis are very positive," Dr. Mandolesi interjects. "This is very exciting to us—to find something that helps multiple sclerosis patients and to do the research that documents the results statistically. The first study was with only eight patients, but our second and current study is with over 500 patients, 370 with MS and 147 in our control group that have non-neurological conditions. We are very excited and encouraged by the results we are getting.

"Working with MS is my specialty," Dr. Mandolesi continued, "and as I have studied MS patients, I have seen a problem with compression of the neck. So it was conceivable to me that changing the position of the neck might improve the MS condition. The C-1 is very important because in front of it, we have the jugular vein. We have studied these patients before and after Upper Cervical Care, using X-rays to see how C-1 had been adjusted and to verify our results. After many such tests, we have scientific proof that the Upper Cervical correction is effective. These patients changed nothing in their care during the study; they only added Upper Cervical Care.

"Our current study will be much more scientifically conclusive and will be published and presented to the medical community. The problem, as I see it, between medical doctors and chiropractors is lack of understanding. At the moment, we are trying to join the two groups through knowledge of this research so when medical doctors ask the question 'Why or how does this help?' we will be able to answer with scientific proof. That is our goal.

"We think that Upper Cervical Care can improve the hemodynamic conditions and clinical symptoms of multiple sclerosis patients," Dr. Mandolesi said. "The preliminary reports show that the entire sample of multiple sclerosis patients has vascular lesions, particularly on vertebral veins; that is the pathway of our interest, along with a misalignment of the C1 (atlas) vertebra. This supports our theory of there being a mechanical postural vascular block in MS patients with chronic cerebrospinal venous insufficiency (CCSVI)."[90]

Each year for the past four years, Dr. Mandolesi and Dr. Marceca have presented their research findings on MS patients under Upper Cervical Care at Evolution, Upper Cervical Health Centers' annual convention. In their 2012 presentation to Upper Cervical doctors, they reported that "MS patients under Upper Cervical Care showed an average reduction of more than 50% of the symptoms attributed to the disease, verified by both X-rays and clinical results, and that based on these findings, it is our belief that Upper Cervical Care should be a primary treatment of the mechanical cause of MS and that there is evidence that Upper Cervical Care can prevent the disease."[91]

Dr. Mandolesi is highly respected in Italy's medical community. His research on the effectiveness of Upper Cervical Care has resulted in an insurgence of MS patients in my Upper Cervical clinic in Rome as medical doctors there have started referring patients to us for care.

Pain: Pain has been defined by the International Association for the Study of Pain as an unpleasant sensory and emotional experience associated with actual or potential tissue damage. Clinical studies have shown Upper Cervical Care effective in the treatment of back, neck, knee, shoulder, and arm pain.

A study by Uri Herzberg hypothesized that chronic pain can influence the immune system.[92] Perhaps that is why patients who come to see Upper Cervical doctors for back pain are often surprised to see their body heal from other diseases, as well.

A case study out of Sweden listed the following symptoms and conditions that can result from cervical spinal cord tension: neck pain, upper extremity pain, numbness and weakness, difficulty in performing fine movements with the hands, lower back pain, lower extremity pain, loss of balance and clumsiness, headaches, shoulder pain, impaired bladder and rectal function, paralysis and spasticity, and respiratory difficulty.[93]

Trigeminal Neuralgia (TN): In a survey of Upper Cervical chiropractors who work with patients suffering from TN, it was found that some patients obtain immediate relief and most patients respond with some relief within two weeks of care. Of the 68 patients with TN, 73.5% received complete relief, 21% obtained some relief, and only 6% were not helped at all with Upper Cervical Care.[94]

Vertigo: A study done by McPartland and Brodeur discussed how cervical spine manipulation has been shown to have a beneficial effect on poor standing balance and vertigo.[95]

In another article, "Vertigo Caused by Disorders of the Cervical Vertebral Column," E. Biesinger discussed how chiropractors are well acquainted with the correlation between the cervical spine dysfunction and the neuro-otological symptoms such as tinnitus, vertigo, neuralgia, and sudden hearing loss.[96]

I have attempted, with this abbreviated list of conditions, to summarize some of the research that supports what we do in Upper Cervical Care. Again, for those looking for more in-depth information, I recommend Dr. Eriksen's book.

✳ ✳ ✳

Cynthia P.,—Upper Cervical Patient
Suffered from migraines

In 1998, I was having two to three full-blown migraines a week. When I wasn't having a migraine, I'd still have a headache. So, I basically lived with a headache every day of my life for seven years. When I had a migraine, I'd often spend all day in bed because I just couldn't function. Some days I'd just push through the pain; other days I'd have to leave work, go home, and go to bed. Some nights I'd go to bed feeling fine, and at two or three o'clock in the morning, I'd wake up with a migraine, just excruciating pain. I couldn't pinpoint anything that might be triggering my migraines.

Once I was suffering with a migraine so bad that my husband took me to the emergency room. Without even X-raying me, the doctor said it sounded like I had a ruptured disk, and he recommended that I see a surgeon, that I probably needed back surgery. Well, I wasn't having any of that.

Usually, I'd go to my family doctor when I had a migraine. The office staff knew when I came in what

I was there for. They took me straight back, put me in a darkened room and gave me a shot. My husband would take me home and put me to bed where I'd stay all day. I couldn't stand for my husband to even touch the sheets on the bed; it would feel like he was moving the whole bed. I had to have total darkness. I was just supersensitive to my surroundings. The next day I'd have this hung-over feeling from the medication I'd taken for the migraine. This scenario played out over and over and over.

One thing that's hard for migraine sufferers is that some people think you're putting on, that you're not really hurting, or I've felt people thinking, oh, well, Cynthia's got a migraine again, whatever. Other migraine patients have told me they've experienced the same thing. Nobody has any idea until they have one because you feel like your head's exploding. One of the scary things for me was the statistics about migraine sufferers being more likely to have a stroke later in life. I knew I had to do something, but I didn't know what.

The doctor I went to for my migraines sent me to a neurologist who did a CAT scan and all kinds of other tests. My dad's mom and his sister had migraines, so the doctor chalked my migraines up to heredity. He told me he could give me medication for it, but that I'd have to learn to live with the fact that I was going to have migraines. The neurologist was going to put me on a seizure medication, and I'm not big on taking prescription meds at all, so that didn't sit well with me. Plus, he told me I'd have to take it every day for the rest of my life, and I thought, no, I'm not doing that.

Then I met a woman at church who had a daughter who suffered from seizures who was coming to Upper Cervical Care. She suggested I go see an Upper Cervical doctor to see if Upper Cervical could help my migraines. I had been going to a full-spine chiropractor with mixed results. Sometimes the adjustments helped; sometimes they didn't.

Before getting my first Upper Cervical adjustment, I'd had a migraine for two weeks that I had not been able to get rid of, even with the medication. Some days I could function, and some days I couldn't.

During the rest period, after my first Upper Cervical adjustment, my head felt like it was going to explode. Then suddenly there was like this rush—at the time I didn't understand what was happening, now I know it was my circulation opening up—it was a physical sensation I felt throughout my body. My face tingled, my cheeks got rosy, and as that rush came in, my headache went away as I was lying there. That was a wow moment. I did not have another migraine from that day in March until the end of June—three months later. In seven years of suffering from migraines, I had never gone that long between headaches.

I kept coming in to be checked and adjusted because Upper Cervical was working for me when nothing else had. I mean, I got immediate relief after seven years of pain. I thought, this is amazing! The night of my first adjustment I went to my doctor's patient orientation class and took my husband with me. The place was packed. My husband admitted later that when I came home all excited telling him my migraine went away after my first

Upper Cervical adjustment, he was skeptical. But after the doctor explained how the nervous system works, my husband decided to get under Upper Cervical Care for his sinus problems. And he got better, too.

During my first year of Upper Cervical Care, I had one migraine every three months. After that first year, and for the last six years, I haven't had a migraine.

I've listened to my doctor talk about how often a long-forgotten trauma experienced by the nervous system can initiate a health condition that becomes chronic years later. Then one day I remembered how, years ago, I hit my tailbone so hard on a water slide that it felt like a surge of electricity going through my body. About six months later, I had my first migraine. I'm convinced that injury resulted in my having migraines.

My advice to people who are considering Upper Cervical Care is to be patient and consistent. Not everybody gets the immediate results I did, but I work in an Upper Cervical office now, and I've seen a lot of patients come and go. Sometimes it works very quickly. Sometimes it works gradually. But it does work. Be patient. Stick with it.

Upper Cervical changed my life. It gave me back my life.

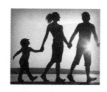

CHAPTER 10

What New Upper Cervical Patients Can Expect

"The only alternative to chiropractic is living a life of less than full expression."

B. J. Palmer

The purpose of this chapter is to answer some of the questions new patients have either verbalized to me or I have sensed they were wondering when they came in for Upper Cervical Care for the first time. Many had already been to numerous doctors and specialists but were not getting better. These patients often fear that Upper Cervical will be just another failed attempt in their effort to get well. Some come in leery of chiropractic in general. Maybe they've been subject to the biased opinion of others; maybe they had a bad experience. Whatever. Their expressions ask: Am I wasting my time here? Am I wasting my money? Can Upper Cervical Care help me? They want desperately to believe that it can, but they're skeptical. After all, they've had their hopes dashed before.

It's normal and natural that patients coming in for a new form of health care feel some trepidation. That's why my office staff and I try to make patients feel at ease every time they come in, but especially during their first office visit. Office procedures and protocol will most certainly vary among Upper Cervical doctors, but there will be some commonalities as well.

On patients' first visit, if they haven't filled out the paperwork we e-mailed them prior to their appointment, they do that upon their arrival. This required paperwork covers the usual: health history, current health challenges, prior surgeries, medications they're currently taking, and information about their insurance. One of my office staff gives new patients a tour of the office. People feel more comfortable knowing where everything is: the restrooms, the play area for children, the X-ray room, the consultation rooms, the adjusting room, and the rest area. Now when they're brought back to me, they'll know what lies behind those closed doors, and hopefully, they'll feel a little more comfortable.

I join new patients in the consultation room where, after introductions, we discuss their current health concerns. I ask if they remember having a fall, injury, or accident, as these are the most common causes of upper cervical subluxations that can result in all kinds of symptoms. I ask patients to tell me about anything that is causing them discomfort.

Then I explain the philosophy of Upper Cervical Care. I tell patients my goal is to see if I can find the cause of the problem they're having, and if I find the cause, I will then explain what I can do to try to fix it. I also tell them if it's something I cannot help them with, I'll try to find them someone who can.

Next, I take new patients to the adjusting room where, using models and charts, I show them how Upper Cervical Care works. My conversation with them goes something like this: "I'm looking for something in your upper cervical area, your neck basically, called a subluxation, a big word for a simple condition. It means that one of the top two bones in your neck could have got misaligned, maybe years ago, to the point that it could have squeezed down on the brain stem, which controls every function of your body. It's like the switchboard operator between your brain and heart, liver, lungs, kidneys, arms, legs—virtually every part and system of your body. The brain stem is the *connector* between the brain and the rest of the body. If either of these upper cervical bones got misaligned to the point it started to compress or put pressure on any area of the brain stem, the pressure would interfere with the pathways that go to a particular part of the body. So wherever those neural pathways were going, that part of the body would not get the full message from the brain, so it would start to malfunction or create symptoms." (I use models of the atlas and axis and another of the nerve fibers going through the brain stem to illustrate as I explain all this.)

"For example, the brain tells the pancreas to produce insulin, so if the misalignment is pressing on the brain stem in the area at which these messages to the pancreas need to flow freely through the brain stem, the messages don't get through, and the pancreas doesn't know to produce the insulin the body needs. Those messages were *interfered with* because one of the upper cervical bones was misaligned. So the first thing I'm looking for is pressure on the brain stem.

"Now, the head sits on top of these upper cervical bones, so anywhere these bones go, the head goes with it. It doesn't have any choice because it sits right on top. The brain sits on top of these two bones encased by the skull, and our brain has to be level to work right. Now, the brain has its own reflex called the righting reflex, and its purpose is just as it sounds, to right itself. Our brain must be balanced or parallel to the ground. If one of these upper cervical bones gets out of alignment, it throws the head out of balance. The brain doesn't like that, and the righting reflex kicks in, telling the brain that it's off balance. The brain responds by sending messages to the body telling the body to compensate or change until the head levels out.

"This can start a chain reaction of twisting, turning, bending, or rotating—whatever the body has to do to get that head level. As a result, you end up with compensatory changes in the neck, upper back, lower back, even in your legs, knees, and feet. With gravity always pushing down, just going through normal motions can cause these compensations to become weak spots, which can turn into neck pain, back pain, arm pain, leg pain, any kind of pain. Therefore, it could be you have a problem in the upper part of your neck that is *causing* the aches and pains in the rest of your body."

"The Law of Demand and Supply is existent in the body in its ideal state; wherein the 'clearing house' is the

brain, Innate the virtuous 'banker,' the brain cells, 'clerks,' and nerve cells, 'messengers.'"

B. J. Palmer

I explain to patients that if they have a subluxation, we'll find several things going on in their upper neck: pain and tenderness, muscle spasms, joint fixation, which means the bones don't move like they're supposed to, and most importantly, heat and/or body imbalance. If you put pressure on a nerve, especially a nerve as big as the brain stem, it's going to get hot, and if one of the Upper Cervical bones gets misaligned, it will throw the head off balance, causing the rest of the body to compensate.

Seventy-five trillion neural pathways run through the brain stem. There is a pathway to and from the brain for every cell in your body, and the body has about 75 trillion cells. Every cell has direct communication to the brain. (Talk about fiber optics!)

Then I show patients two drawings—one that shows the head and neck aligned, a body in balance, and another drawing that shows the atlas out of alignment.

I explain that when the head is tilted, the whole body is out of balance. I use these pictures to illustrate what I told them earlier: that the brain doesn't like being out of balance, so it sends messages to the body to compensate or change until the head gets level. The body might pull one shoulder down or pull one hip up, making one leg shorter than the other. So the person whose upper cervical is out of alignment ends up stretched or contracted, with tight muscles in the neck, upper back, lower back, maybe even in the hamstrings or calves. The body compensates however it can to get the head level. However, this compensation, over time, can result in neck pain, shoulder pain, leg pain, back pain, knee pain, etc.

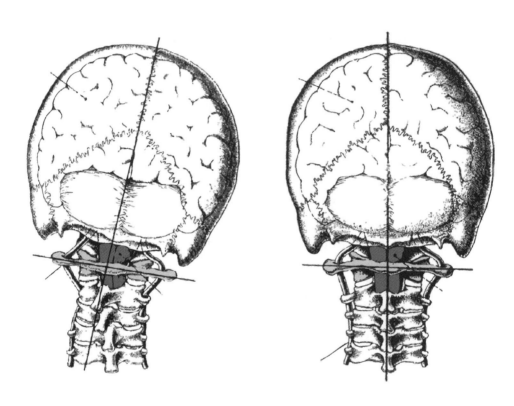

Reprinted with permission of Daniel O. Clark, DC
www.uppercervicalillustrations.com

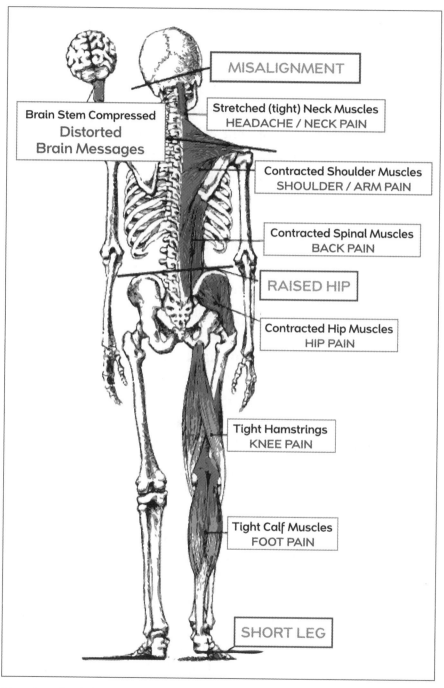

MISALIGNMENT

Brain Stem Compressed
Distorted
Brain Messages

Stretched (tight) Neck Muscles
HEADACHE / NECK PAIN

Contracted Shoulder Muscles
SHOULDER / ARM PAIN

Contracted Spinal Muscles
BACK PAIN

RAISED HIP

Contracted Hip Muscles
HIP PAIN

Tight Hamstrings
KNEE PAIN

Tight Calf Muscles
FOOT PAIN

SHORT LEG

Reprinted with permission of Daniel O. Clark, DC
www.uppercervicalillustrations.com

Biomechanically, our bodies are designed to resist the pull of gravity perpendicular. If one leg gets pulled up, it throws everything off. Think of a car. If your car got out of alignment, and instead of taking it to the shop to get an alignment, you just kept driving it, driving it, driving it—eventually, parts of that car are going to wear out. The longer you keep driving it, the more parts are going to wear down. Your body reacts the same way unless it is realigned. If you hit a curve or drive over potholes, it's going to throw your car out of alignment. If your body is subject to physical, emotional, or chemical stress—and all bodies are—it can misalign one of the bones in the upper neck and cause compensatory misalignments throughout your body, as well. Upper Cervical misalignments need to be realigned for optimal performance.

It is usually at this point that I sit down with patients and talk specifically about the two upper cervical bones, the only two vertebrae about which I'm concerned. Using a hand-held model, I point to the first bone of the neck, the atlas, called that because it holds up the "world," which, in this case, is their head. The second cervical bone is called the axis because our world pivots here. In fact, the atlas-axis articulation is the only pivot joint and the most freely movable joint in the body. Because there are no bony locks to hold it, the atlas can slide, it can turn, and it can go up and down.

The computer device I use to check for pressure on the brain stem is called a TyTron. It has two probes that measure heat. I roll the TyTron up the patient's neck, an entirely painless process, and the TyTron measures and compares the temperature on each side of the patient's neck. I start at the seventh cervical and roll it up to the base of the skull. The body is symmetrical. That means the temperature should be the same on both sides. But if one of the bones in the neck is misaligned to the point that it is putting pressure on the brain stem, that area will get hot, and we'll see that in the form of a line graph on the monitor. If one side of the neck is hotter than the other side, I know there's some kind of pressure there.

Technology has come a long way since the days of B. J. Palmer, who developed the Upper Cervical technique in his then state-of-the-art research laboratory. Upper Cervical doctors today use a variety of sophisticated tools to evaluate patients as well as different techniques to adjust. They all work.

I show patients what a perfect alignment looks like compared to theirs as measured by the TyTron. During this first exam, I get a sense of the patient's pattern. Everyone has a unique pattern when the bone is out of alignment. In Upper Cervical, we often refer to this pattern as the patient's "sick pattern."

Many Upper Cervical doctors will check for body imbalance by doing a posture analysis. This is achieved by looking for head tilt, low shoulder, high hip, and ultimately having the patient lie down and measure leg length to determine if one leg is shorter than the other. If body imbalance and/or the TyTron exam revealed that the patient's upper cervical bones are out of alignment, I discuss with him/her the importance of X-rays.

There are 274 ways C1 and C2, the atlas and axis, can misalign. I use a digital X-ray that is laser aligned and has an L-frame, which means it's guaranteed for life to be perfectly aligned. The laser ensures that it lines up exactly on the crosshairs so that it is perpendicular. Even the slightest angle would create a shadow that could change the X-ray reading. These X-rays are as close to perfect as we can currently get. That's important because the exact measurement of the misalignment, which allows Upper Cervical doctors to make a more exact correction, is what makes Upper Cervical *specific chiropractic*. A fraction of a degree can be the difference in someone getting better or not. I take three X-rays—one from the side, one from the front, and one from underneath—so we'll have a three-dimensional view of the atlas and axis and how the patient is aligned or out of alignment. Some Upper Cervical techniques might require more X-ray views. *All* Upper Cervical doctors take X-rays because the X-ray shows us exactly what we need to do to correct the misalignment.

That's the end of a patient's first visit with me. Since there are 274 ways the atlas and axis can be misaligned, I need time to sit down and study the X-rays—to measure, mark, and draw angles, to determine exactly how those two bones are out of alignment.

On the patient's second visit, I review his/her X-rays, this time showing the patient the exact misalignment that I'll be correcting. I again check the patient with the TyTron to help establish his/her particular pattern or fingerprint. I want to know what his/her pattern looks like when the patient is misaligned because he/she is going to produce the same pattern every time he/she is out of alignment. (Some patients have their pattern printed out and take it with them.) Some Upper Cervical doctors will reevaluate the patient for body imbalance, looking for consistent findings to establish a postural pattern to determine when the patient will need to be adjusted in the future.

Next, I give the patient an Upper Cervical adjustment (which does not hurt). After the adjustment, the patient lies down in a room created just for that purpose. Resting for 15 to 20 minutes immediately following an adjustment helps the adjustment hold. Remember, in Upper Cervical, *holding is healing.* Usually, resting in a darkened room, listening to healing music, is the Upper Cervical patient's favorite time during the appointment.

After the resting period, the patient is again checked with the TyTron to see if the lines on the monitor are straight, which would reflect that the nerve pressure has been removed and the subluxation corrected. Some doctors will also check the patient to determine whether the postural imbalances have been corrected.

I tell the patient that the key now is to keep that bone where it is. Any kind of stress—physical, emotional, even chemical stress—can pull it back into its familiar, pre-adjustment misalignment. For the body to start healing, the adjustment must hold. I go over ways patients can minimize stress to the upper cervical area, which basically requires that they be aware of ways they're using their neck that might bring stress to the area. (Don't paint any ceilings when you're in the early stages of Upper Cervical Care. Don't hold the phone with your chin and shoulder. Don't sleep on your stomach—on the side is okay, but on the back is ideal, provided you don't prop your head up with a bunch of pillows.)

It's also important that patients stay well-hydrated, especially in the beginning, as their body will be going through some changes during the healing process. Their posture is going to shift; they're going to build up lactic acid because they're going to start using muscles that have been on vacation. Water will help flush out the lactic acid. Sometimes when the body starts to heal, it detoxes, so I explain to patients that they might feel a little yucky at first. This is nothing to be concerned about. It's part of the healing process, and again, water will help keep the body flushed out.

I send new patients home with a water bottle and a pamphlet on the Do's and Don'ts after an Upper Cervical Adjustment as a reminder because I realize I have given them a lot of information that most have never heard before.

On the patient's third visit, I check him/her again with the TyTron and do an adjustment, if needed (but only if needed). Then I go over a report, which I have created just for that patient, which he/she gets a copy of. Each Upper Cervical Care Plan is based on the patient's particular condition and imminent needs. I consider factors such as the patient's age, what the X-rays have shown us, what we know (if anything) about the precipitating cause, the severity of the symptoms, how long the patient has had the condition, and how the patient responded to the first Upper Cervical adjustment.

My recommendation is based on the data from his/her two prior appointments plus my experience dealing with patients with similar conditions. I explain to patients that I expect each Upper Cervical adjustment to hold longer and longer, which means they'll need to see me less and less. However, in the beginning it's very important that as soon as the bone goes out that we're there to put it back in; the quicker the body accepts the correct alignment, the quicker the patient will get better. I remind patients that the upper cervical spine is subject to strain during everyday life and that not only is it possible that their correction recede toward the old, abnormal position, necessitating another correction until the new correction finally holds, but often, tissues that have, perhaps for years, assumed an abnormal condition due to pressure on the nerve fibers must be rebuilt in order for the vertebra to hold the "new normal" position.

At this time, I usually explain the three phases of the healing process. The first is the intensive or acute phase. This phase can be a bit of a roller coaster ride for the patient. I tell patients there will be times when they feel better, and there will be times they don't feel so well. They might feel like they're bouncing back and forth until they get to a point that they'll start having more and more good days and fewer and fewer bad days, until eventually, they can forget about the bad days.

Healing is a very individual process. Every Upper Cervical doctor has had patients who have one or two adjustments and—bam!—their symptoms disappear for good! We love it when that happens, but it's certainly not everybody's experience, so I'd rather underestimate and over deliver. Most patients start experiencing this time of *more good days than bad days* after being under Upper Cervical Care for two to four weeks. For some, it comes earlier than that, and for a few, it comes later. The time it takes for patients to heal does not always equal the time it took for the symptoms to develop. As a general rule, however, acute conditions respond rapidly, while chronic, long-standing cases may be slower to respond.

The second phase of healing is the corrective stage. This is when patients start to notice an improvement in their overall health. Most patients start to notice that they are sleeping better; they have more energy; their immune system is getting stronger; their digestion starts to normalize. These improvements happen regardless of the condition for which they sought Upper Cervical Care.

"As it took time for the condition to change from health to a maximum degree of abnormality, it takes time to retrace back to health."

B. J. Palmer

The last phase of healing is the rehabilitation or strengthening phase. At this point, I might give patients some light exercises to help them strengthen the muscles in their neck and back to give them more stability. Our goal is to get patients' appointments down to one per month. I have some patients that can hold their adjustments for three to six months, but most need to be checked every month to six weeks. This is our Wellness Program.

Halfway through the patient's Upper Cervical Care Plan, I will take new X-rays to see where we are, like you'd check a road map to see where you are in relation to your destination. It also provides a snapshot of the progress we've made. We look at the changes the Upper Cervical corrections have made in the neck, and if there's anything we need to tweak, we do it here. We don't want to get to the end and realize we missed something and have to go back and correct it.

It is also during that third appointment that I schedule patients for our Patient Orientation Class, which I require all new patients attend. The class lasts about an hour, maybe a little longer if patients have a lot of questions. I believe for patients to get the most out of their Upper Cervical Care Plan it is very important that they come to the orientation class because I cover things they need to understand about Upper Cervical Care that I don't have time to discuss during an office visit.

I promise patients that I will talk about things they probably have never heard before and won't hear anywhere else that are very important to their health. I encourage patients to bring someone to the orientation class who cares about them, their spouse if they're married, so their loved one can understand what's going on with their health and what they'll be going through to get it restored. Everyone is welcome to our classes. Our patients often refer their friends and family to our classes to learn more about Upper Cervical Care. I have had vanloads of people drive several hours to attend the orientation class.

One of the things I cover at my Patient Orientation Class that I have not yet written about in this book is the phenomenon called retracing. Retracing is the re-experiencing or re-awakening of old symptoms, including pain, memories, and even emotions, during the healing process. Every single experience you've had in your life is stored in your central nervous system. Sometimes symptoms that have not manifested for months or even years will reoccur.

Even though such experiences are part of the healing process, many people confuse them with an exacerbation of their current state of health when, in fact, nothing could be further from the truth. Retracing is a 100% natural phenomenon. It occurs in holistic healing disciplines when body balance and homeostasis (both internally and externally) are reestablished.

Healing responses are little understood in the medical profession, because they rarely occur with drug therapy. Drugs either inhibit or stimulate bodily functions as opposed to restoring health. The body learns to adapt to the problem rather than heal through it. As a result, most people, including medical doctors, are usually unfamiliar with them. However, anyone who comes under Upper Cervical Care may experience retracing to some degree.

I have had patients share with me that while they were lying in the resting area following their Upper Cervical adjustment, without provocation, they started laughing, or crying, or thinking of things they hadn't thought about for years. Emotional and psychological healing responses are among the most interesting and often most important. I always tell patients they should welcome such occurrences because they indicate their body is healing, even if it might make them feel a little weird at the time.

Sometimes patients discontinue their care prematurely when they start retracing because it makes them feel uncomfortable. This is a mistake. They could be denying themselves a complete healing experience. Most healing responses are mild and pass very quickly; I'd say typically, retracing lasts from one day to a couple of weeks. I always tell patients to share with me what they're experiencing while under Upper Cervical Care, whether they're feeling like a million bucks or absolutely awful, but to rest assured that as long as their corrections are holding, they are healing. Patience, always a virtue, is especially important as the body retraces its way back to health.

I give patients a copy of the Upper Cervical Care Plan that we just discussed and let one of my office staff talk to them about the cost of the plan, what their insurance will pay, and the different payment options available to them. I hear stories from patients all the time about how they were shocked to get medical bills in the mail for hundreds, sometimes thousands of dollars. They had no idea what these costs were going to be when they left the doctor's office. Most people, including yours truly, like to know what they're committing to financially before they make a decision, so I tell my patients upfront what the cost of their Upper Cervical Care Plan will be, how much they can expect their insurance or Medicare to pay, and the options they have for paying the balance, if there is one.

Compared to the cost of drugs and surgery, I think Upper Cervical Care is the best bargain in health care. I'm sure the patients whose stories you've been reading would tell you that, for them, Upper Cervical Care was a good investment.

I'm reminded of a patient who came to me during my first year in practice when I was still wet behind the ears but already confident that Upper Cervical Care could help everyone, regardless of their condition. This female patient—we'll call her Mrs. Jones—had been referred to me by a friend.

Mrs. Jones told me that she had spent over $180,000 trying to get pregnant. She had been to the Mayo Clinic. She had been to Duke University and Johns Hopkins. She had been to the best fertility clinic in Atlanta. Her dream was to have a child, and according to her, she had been everywhere and tried everything, but nothing had worked. I could tell Mrs. Jones was thinking that she was wasting her time with me, a 25-year-old who had just hung out his shingle on his little 600-square-foot, paneled office in small-town, North Carolina.

So I told Mrs. Jones what I tell all my patients: "Sometimes the upper two bones of the neck can be misaligned and therefore interfere with the normal transmission of nerve energy from your brain to other parts of the body—in your case, the reproductive system. If that communication is interfered with, the reproductive system doesn't work as it was intended to work. If the reproductive system isn't working properly, no matter what you do externally, your body will not be able to create and develop a child. But if we can open up those messages from the brain to the reproductive system, allowing the reproductive system to work the way it's designed to work, then the messages can normalize and the chances of your ability to produce the egg and to nurture the embryo into a child are greatly improved. Now what I can do—all I can do—is to look at you and determine if you have a blockage in the mental impulse from the brain to the reproductive system. If I can find it, I can correct it, then everything else is up to God."

"Well, I don't know how you can help me. I've been to the best of the best and they couldn't help me. But I'm here," Mrs. Jones sighed, "let's just do it."

So I took X-rays and checked her neck with a derma-thermograph, which tells me if there's a blockage between the brain and the body, and we found a blockage. I showed her the blockage on the X-rays and made a specific correction of the first bone in her neck, then did another scan to make sure the blockage was removed. It was removed.

I told Mrs. Jones that I would need to check her periodically over the next six months because we had to make sure the pressure stayed off her brain stem, thus allowing the full mental capacity from the brain to get to the reproductive system continuously. Over time, her reproductive system should normalize and increase her chances of having a child.

"Well," Mrs. Jones replied, "we might as well forget this because I'm moving to Dallas in a month. I can't be here for six months."

"Okay," I answered, "let's give it a month and see what happens. Over the next month, I'll check you periodically to see if that bone is holding the adjustment. If it is, we leave it alone. If it's slipped out of alignment, we'll put it back in again."

Mrs. Jones agreed, walked out, and never came back.

A couple of months later, my front desk assistant told me I had a phone call.

"Is this Dr. Drury?" a faintly familiar voice asked.

"Yes, it is," I replied.

"I L-O-V-E you, Dr. Drury," a voice I now recognized as Mrs. Jones's was shouting with joy. "Remember me? I came to see you after spending $180,000 traveling all over the country to see fertility specialists. You adjusted my neck one time. I didn't even come back when I told you I would, and now I'm pregnant! The only thing I did differently these last two months was come see you. So thank you! I can't tell you how happy we are! You've given me something I was beginning to think I'd never have, and I'm so appreciative."

"You're very welcome," I answered, "and I wish you and the baby the best."

When I hung up the phone, I was almost as excited as Mrs. Jones. I had to tell somebody, so I called Mom.

"Mom!" I blurted out as soon as she said hello. "Guess what? I got a lady pregnant!"

Long pause. Finally, my mom said, weakly, "Ray, you're talking about a patient who came to you for an infertility problem, right?"

Later that evening, I went back and looked at Mrs. Jones's chart. She had spent all that money trying to get pregnant and it never happened. Her total bill with me, including the X-rays, was $210. I think Mrs. Jones would say Upper Cervical Care was a great deal for her.

In Upper Cervical Care, we see patients like Mrs. Jones all the time—people who have spent thousands and thousands of dollars and years of their lives seeking healing and relief from pain. Sadly, many of the patients who come to Upper Cervical do so as a last resort. They come to us after they've exhausted the options offered by traditional medicine and have only a slim hope of ever getting better.

Fortunately, that's enough.

To find the Upper Cervical doctor nearest you, please visit www.BestKeptSecretInHealthCare.com.

✳ ✳ ✳

Linda W.,—Upper Cervical Patient
Sciatica and other pain

I worked as a general chiropractor until injuries from a car accident forced me into early retirement. This and other accidents, which occurred over a period of time, resulted in my having multiple health problems. I had sciatica so bad I couldn't sit for long. Once I was in a car, I had difficulty getting out. I thought if I can't drive, I can't do anything. I also suffered from fibromyalgia and neck pain, but it was the sciatica that was interfering most with my life.

Having been a chiropractor, I knew about the different chiropractic techniques, and I tried most of them, but nothing seemed to help. At the time I heard about Upper Cervical, I was considering back surgery; I was so desperate for relief. Upper Cervical wasn't really taught at the chiropractic college I attended, so I didn't know much about it. But when I saw an ad in the paper about Upper Cervical Care, I decided to go hear this man speak. That was eight years ago.

Soon after I got under Upper Cervical Care, problems I hadn't even told the doctor about went away. For example, I'd had chronic constipation since I was a child, and I'm now in my sixties. Under Upper Cervical Care the constipation went away after my first few adjustments. It took about three months to get the sciatica healed, but because of the other positive changes I was experiencing, I continued with Upper Cervical Care. I mean, after the second or third adjustment, I knew my body was changing. I was just feeling better. For example, I'd always had cracking in my jaw, and that went away. Next, the head and neck pain cleared out. But when what I call this shawl-like pain (because it, like, wrapped around my shoulders), when that went away, I thought, wow. Then the burning and numbness I was having in my fingers—so bad that it would wake me up sometimes—that went away.

But again, it was the sciatica that was interfering with my life. I realized symptoms were going away slowly, from the top down. The doctor kept telling me to be patient, to give it time, that the body had its own way of healing, and sure enough, the sciatica went away, too.

Besides eliminating the pain I was having, Upper Cervical has given me the confidence that I can manage and maintain my health. I don't have to wait for the inevitable surgery or live the rest of my life on prescription drugs. I knew better than to start down the road of taking high-powered meds for the pain; some people get addicted to pain medication and totally mess up their life on a different level. However, when I came to Upper Cervical, I was taking ibuprofen, three or four at a time, and I knew I couldn't continue to do that either.

I was a chemical engineer before I became a chiropractor, and I see many parallels between engineering and the body, the science behind the body's structural component, the complexity of its chemical components, how everything's connected, how one thing affects another— engineering gave me a framework for understanding and appreciating chiropractic.

If you look at neurology, the brain stem is the major moderator of pain. Knowing that, everyone should be looking to deal with pain issues through brain stem involvement, which is what Upper Cervical Care does. I know some people have wow experiences when they come under Upper Cervical Care in that they get almost immediate and lasting relief, a kind of miraculous healing. It wasn't like that for me with my sciatica, but relief did come. I'm still under regular Upper Cervical Care eight years later, because for me, it's been about being able to manage and maintain without fear—and that's important because the medical model is based on fear, and it's great to know that although my body is aging, I don't have to live in fear.

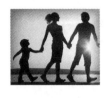

CHAPTER 11

The Ultimate Wellness Program

"Chiropractic is health insurance. Premiums small. Dividends large."

B. J. Palmer

It is easier to stay well than to get well, and the benefits of Upper Cervical Care are not limited by the age of the patient. Dr. Michael Wagner, an Upper Cervical doctor, shared in the documentary, *The Power of Upper Cervical*, that the youngest patient he had adjusted was three hours old and the oldest, 94 years old.

Regular chiropractic care is essential for maintaining the health of the nervous system. Nerve irritations are often present long before symptoms; therefore, spinal care for the entire family is as important as regular medical or dental appointments.

The brain and spinal cord develop in the fetus *first*. That alone should be a clue as to their importance. As stated many times in this book, every organ, system, and cell of the body is controlled by the nervous system. It may be the lungs that exchange oxygen for carbon dioxide, but it is the nervous system that tells the body how to do this. Life energy flows through every cell, all 75 trillion of them, and this flow of energy is coordinated by the nervous system. Common sense should tell us a healthy nerve supply is a prerequisite for a healthy body.

The spine is the central support structure of the body, and the upper cervical spine is the most vulnerable part of that structure. It carries the neurological lifeline from the brain to all other parts of the body. The functional health of the body depends on the flow of an unrestricted nerve system. When your spine suffers, your overall health suffers, too.

"In the future, chiropractic will be valued for its preventative qualities as much as its restorative qualities."

B. J. Palmer

It's very simple. If the brain can't communicate with some part of the body, we're going to get sick, but when the brain *is* fully communicating with all parts of the body, we stay well. Regular Upper Cervical checkups ensure that the upper cervical bones, the atlas and axis, are in alignment, which means that the neural canal, the brain stem, is clear, which allows Innate Intelligence, that in-born wisdom that we all have, to flow from above-down, inside-out, and that is what restores and maintains health.

Chiropractic care is not a replacement for medical care, but a separate and distinct profession that provides a unique health care service. Upper Cervical chiropractors detect and correct subluxations in the upper cervical area to reduce neurological interference, which helps patients achieve optimum health, regardless of the patient's symptoms or conditions.

We do not treat patients for conditions. *Whatever* the patient is suffering from, if the body can get back to normal functioning, healing will happen. Innate Intelligence, which travels via the nervous system, animates the body and regulates the healing process.

When you make Upper Cervical Care part of your wellness program, you are giving your body its best chance to be as healthy as possible and to *not have* chronic pain, illnesses, diseases, or ailments later in life. Health is much more than being disease-free. As the adage goes, if you don't take care of you health, it will go away, and if you don't take care of your body, where will you live?

It is very frustrating for Upper Cervical doctors—and this happens a lot—to see patients regain their health under Upper Cervical Care, then disappear. Almost always, these patients are back in our clinics a few months or years later, in pain, dealing with all kinds of symptoms, that they would've never had if they'd had regular checkups as maintenance. Regular checkups are the only way to ensure that health problems get corrected and symptoms do not return.

Remember, in Upper Cervical, holding is healing. Upper Cervical doctors do not adjust patients if our testing instruments show us they are holding the adjustment. If we were to make a correction when it isn't necessary, it could actually slow down the healing process and potentially cause more problems. Upper Cervical doctors are *very* conservative when it comes to making corrections. However, we don't know if a patient is holding the adjustment unless we check him or her periodically. Just as people's bodies heal differently, bodies don't hold adjustments for the same length of time.

As Upper Cervical doctors, we initially check patients to see if they have an upper cervical subluxation. If they do, we adjust their atlas and axis, the two upper cervical bones, then check to make sure they are in alignment. *Then we get out of the way,* continue to monitor the patient, and let healing happen. Once patients have had their health restored, we put them on a maintenance program to make sure their upper cervical bones *stay* in alignment and to make a correction if, and only if, they slip out of alignment. That's how patients maintain their newly restored health. An Upper Cervical wellness program is the key to *staying* well.

Upper Cervical Care is not a panacea, but it *is* a highly effective health care system that has helped millions of people and can help many millions more. Upper Cervical doctors witness health being restored to patients day in and day out, many who had been told nothing more could be done for them, that they'd just have to learn to live with their health problem. To that, Upper Cervical doctors want to shout, "We do *not* believe you have to live with a debilitating condition, and you owe it to yourself to see if Upper Cervical Care can help you."

In this country, we have been programmed to think of health care as drugs and surgery, which has created a populace who, by and large, know how to be good medical patients. We've all been subjected to the media campaigns that have impacted our attitudes toward health, commercials that show us what health looks like and how to get it. And we've bought it, to the extent that many of us are willing to overlook the list of harmful, sometimes fatal, side effects of some prescription drugs.

Pharmaceutical companies have very deep pockets; they can and do make billions of dollars on a single drug. The financial damage that comes from lawsuits after thousands have had adverse effects taking some of these drugs is a pittance compared to the profits the companies had already made on them.

Let me ask you: "Is there any reason to think drug companies will do anything differently in the near future? It's your health we're talking about. Yes, drugs are sometimes necessary, but medications will not make you healthy.

Dr. Susan Brown-Hooper is an Upper Cervical doctor with a PhD in pharmaceutics. Before Upper Cervical, she worked for 20 years doing research in pharmaceutical science and was very much into the medical model, taking antibiotics for this and pain medication for that. She said that after she started studying alternative health care, it felt strange to realize that methods to help the body heal naturally, like Upper Cervical Care, were there all along, and she just didn't know about them.

There are life-saving drugs out there, but why are we prescribing medications without checking the nervous system first? We're not being told to look at the body to help balance it; we're being told to take another pill, which has side effects.

Surgery is also sometimes necessary, but, again, who would choose surgery before checking out a non-invasive health care procedure like Upper Cervical to see if surgery could be avoided, to see if the body might be able to heal itself naturally?

Let's take an easy example. Eight out of ten people have low back pain at some point in their lives. It's one of the most expensive health care problems in America, *and* it happens to be one that most people, even the skeptics, will say chiropractic might be able to help. Back problems cost this country over $20 billion a year for medical care, and an additional $50 billion in lost productivity. Upper-respiratory ailments are the number one reason most people go to the doctor; back pain is the number two reason. Low back surgery is the third most common surgery performed in the United States, after cesarean section.[97] The cost for lumbar disc surgery can range from $90,000-$140,000.[98] You don't have to be an Einstein (or an economist) to realize it might be worth checking out a safer, much, much, much, much less expensive procedure like Upper Cervical before signing up for back surgery.

"If I'd known I was going to live this long, I'd taken better care of myself."

Mickey Mantle

In an ideal world, all the healing professions would learn about each other's practices and understand the advantages of each approach. I believe that many of the neurologists who have patients who have not been helped under the medical model would refer those patients to Upper Cervical Care if they knew about us.

I want people to know that there are *choices* to be made in health care, choices they can make for themselves, and that Upper Cervical Care should be on that list of choices. It is a safe and effective health care option and a very cost-effective one. Chiropractic has proven itself in principle and practice; its philosophy, science, and art are realistic and factual. Evidence that Upper Cervical Care works has been documented in both clinical trials and double-blind studies.

To turn our health care system around, we as a country have to change the way we think about health, a difficult but not impossible task. Everyone needs to know that there is hope and there is help beyond drugs and surgery. We have to begin thinking that health is natural, and disease is unnatural. (Because it is.) We are *not* fundamentally flawed, and it is *not* true that as we get older, we have to expect things to go wrong with us. Nor do we have to be victims of genetics or environment. What if we believed instead that we are fundamentally perfect, that our bodies have the ability to heal or recover from almost anything? What if we had a health care system that empowered us to seek advice, then make our own decisions? After all, don't we know what is ultimately best for us, really?

Intervention and non-interference. Real simple ideas. If I have a cavity in a tooth, I need an intervention, but for health in general, I need to find out what's keeping my life from working and get that *out* of my life. I need to remove what's interfering with my body's normal, healthy functioning.

In the documentary *The Power of Upper Cervical*, Dr. Robert Brooks relates three enemies of progress to Upper

Cervical Health Care: (1) ignorance—not knowing Upper Cervical Care exists; (2) prejudice—believing something that isn't true, believing the lies that have been spread about chiropractic by the American Medical Association and others; and (3) superstition—fearing the unknown, which keeps you from investigating something that can really help you.

If you have read this book, you are no longer uninformed about Upper Cervical Care. I've also tried to present the facts about chiropractic in a historical context to help dispel some of the myths and prejudices that have maligned the profession from its inception. If you're still a bit superstitious, meaning you have a fear of the unknown that might keep you from investigating something like Upper Cervical, I don't know how to help you, other than to suggest that you read more patient testimonials in the Appendix, or go to our website at UpperCervicalCare.com and view some of the dozens of Upper Cervical patients' stories on video.

At the end of my Patient Orientation Class, I used to say, "Now that you have this information, I hope you will share it with someone you know who is sick or suffering." I don't say that anymore. There are too many people who *are* sick and suffering, loaded up on medication or preparing for unnecessary surgery. Instead, I say, "Now that you have this information, you have a *responsibility* to share it with someone you know who is sick or suffering." Information by itself is not power; it's what you do with information that can be powerful.

I hope something you have read in *The Best-Kept Secret in Health Care* becomes a powerful force for good in your, or a loved one's, life. To find an Upper Cervical doctor near you, visit www.BestKeptSecretInHealthCare.com.

* * *

Bill and Jan K., *Upper Cervical Patients*

My wife and I were driving by and saw Specific Chiropractic on a sign, and I said to my wife, "Wonder what that is?" I'd been to a lot of chiropractors, and I was curious, so I decided to make an appointment. That was almost 20 years ago when my Upper Cervical doc first opened his practice. When he moved his office to over an hour away from us, we drove there, so we could keep seeing him. Upper Cervical helped me in a way other chiropractors and sports medicine doctors didn't. I'm a whole lot better now than I was before I started with Upper Cervical.

When I first came to Upper Cervical, I had all kinds of pain in my joints and muscles—facial pain, neck and shoulder pain, back pain to my waist. My whole left side was just deteriorating. My jaw got broken 30 years ago, and I've had different injuries throughout my life that, I think, caused me pain later on. I rode motorcycles and had a few wrecks; I'm sure that contributed. When I was 35, I was diagnosed with arthritis in my neck. They told me I had the neck of a 60-year-old man.

I always kept on working, but it was tough. I didn't take a lot of prescriptions because I wasn't much into that. Seems like medical doctors burn, cut, or write prescriptions, and that's about it. So I self-medicated with a lot of over-the-counter pain killers and just tried to deal with it, which I know wasn't good for me either. My wife had to deal with it, too, maybe more than me. Being in pain all the time affects your attitude, and not in a positive way.

One thing I liked was that the doctor spent a lot of time explaining Upper Cervical and how it worked. He was honest to say that since I'd been dealing with my aches and pain for years, this would probably not be a quick fix, and it wasn't. Whenever he told me something, I'd find myself saying to myself, "Well, that makes sense. That makes sense. That makes sense." So I decided to give it a try, and I'm really glad I did. About six to eight weeks into treatment, I knew I was feeling better. I was having less pain. That's why all these years later, I still come in for regular checkups. I don't want to get back in the shape I was when I first came to Upper Cervical.

I tell other people about Upper Cervical all the time, but if I have anything to say to people seeking Upper Cervical Care, it is that they should give it time. The body does have the ability to heal, but just like my injuries and the pain from them happened to me over time, that's how I experienced healing, over time. I was so messed up, my healing came slow. I knew that it took years for me to get where I was, so I didn't expect to be pain-free in 30 days, although after a few weeks I was feeling a whole lot better.

People give up too soon. I've seen people I've referred come one time but not come back, and I think, why? Everybody's looking for a quick fix. We're used

*to microwave ovens, drive-through restaurants; every-
thing is now, now, now. Healing doesn't usually work
that way.*

*I'm just happy I've been able to maintain the healing
I've experienced with Upper Cervical, and I think it's
because I come in for regular checkups. My neck is not
nearly as fused as it was; my range of motion is incredible compared to what it used to be, although the doctor
had a heck of a time getting me to loosen up. There's no
doubt in my mind that Upper Cervical Care works. I
do believe that Upper Cervical focuses on getting to the
root of the problem from the brain stem down. What the
Upper Cervical doctor does with the upper neck takes
care of the whole body.*

*Most people know chiropractors, but they don't know
anything about Upper Cervical chiropractic. That's what
they need to know about. True cases of people who have
been helped always influenced me. I've seen a lot of those
cases right here in this office. I don't have anything to
gain by saying this; I just want people who are hurting
to know about Upper Cervical. And again, I want them
to know they're going to have to stick with it long enough
to give it a chance to work. I recall my doctor talking
about retracing, how the first symptoms you had become
the last to leave your body. That's how it worked for me.*

*The basic, common-sense approach to things always
works best with me. When I understood how that atlas
and axis work together and how if you keep those aligned,
the nerves can flow like they're supposed to so the body
can do what it's supposed to—heal itself—like I said, it
made sense, and it worked for me.*

"I like how the doctor scans your neck before the adjustment and shows you where you're out of alignment," Jan, his wife, added, *"then after he adjusts you and you've rested, he brings you back in to show you how the bones are now more aligned after the adjustment. You can actually see your progress; you can see the correction on the computer screen."*

"Most people want a quick, medical fix," Jan added, and Bill nodded in agreement. *"They go to the doctor, get a prescription, and if that doesn't work, they try another one. That's how most people think."*

"As I understand it, Upper Cervical focuses on the electrical current that has to flow through our bodies for everything to function the way it's supposed to. The brain controls all that current like a circuit breaker box does in your house," Bill interjected. *"That's how I think of it. Like I said, keep it simple. It works."*

"And like Bill said," Jan added, *"Stick with it. Even if you don't feel like going in for a checkup. Go. Even if you have to drive like we do. My older sister was being helped by Upper Cervical, but she stopped going, because it was an hour-and-a-half drive, one way. I say keep going, even if you have to drive a distance. It's worth it."*

APPENDIX A

Celebs Who Love Chiropractic

"If it were not for chiropractic, I would not have won the gold medal."

Dan O'Brien, 1996 Decathlon Gold Medalist

A survey commissioned by Landmark Health showed that one in six U.S. adults uses chiropractic services. Check out the celebs who see, or in some cases, *saw* the value of chiropractic care.[99]

Adam Arkin	Air Supply's Graham Russell
Alabama (Band)	Alan Thicke
Alberto Juantorena	Alec Baldwin
Alex Karras	Amy Alcott
Andre Agassi	Barbara Bunkowsky
Baron Davis	Barry Bonds
Bernard Horn	Beth Daniel
Bill Fralic	Bob Christian
Bob Cummings	Bob Hayes
Andy Griffith	Andy Roddick
Anthony Robbins	Arnold Schwarzenegger

"I have been a great devotee of chiropractic my whole life. My father was a medical doctor who stayed well using chiropractic."

Bob Cummings

Atlanta Falcons Team	Brian Boitano
Bruce Jenner	Bruce Willis
Brent Steiner	Byron Hanspard
Burt Reynolds	Candace Pert, PhD
Carol Lawrence	Caruso
Cathy Turner	Charles Barkley
Charles Haley	Cher
Chris Sabo	Christie Brinkley
Chuck Connors	Clarence Darrow
Clifta Coulter	Clint Eastwood
Clint Walker	Connie Smith
Corey Louchiey	Craig Sauer
Crawford Ker	Dallas Cowboys team
Damone Johnson	Dan Marino
Dan Schayes	Daniela Buson
David Cassidy	David Copperfield
David Duchovney	David Spade
Demi Moore	Dammone Johnson
Dennis Weaver	Denver Broncos team
Denzel Washington	Derrick Rose
Detroit Lions team	Detroit Red Wings team
Dianne Carroll	Dixie Carter
Doc Severinsen	Dolph Lundgren
Donna White	Donovan Bailey
Doris Day	Dr. Joyce Vedral

"I am walking today because of chiropractic care I received years ago. I predict a great future for the science of chiropractic."

Jeane Dixon

Dr. Norman Vincent Peale

Ed "Too Tall" Jones

Edwin Moses

Evander Holyfield

Fred Klaven

Gary Clark

George Angat

Gerald Wilkins

Grace Lewis

Heidi Kling

Jack Dempsey

Jack Sikma

James Earl Jones

Jane Russell

Janet Jackson

Jeane Dixon

Jerry Rice

Jerry Seinfeld

Joe Greene

Joe Morgan

Joel Thompson

John DeFendis

John Smoltz

Jonathan Lipnicki

Dwight Stones

Eddie Cantor

Emmitt Smith

Fred Funk

Fred Schneider

Gary Downs

George Kennedy

Golden State Warriors

Greg Matthews

Irving Fryar

Jack LaLanne

James Arness

Jan Stephenson

Jane Seymour

Jason Statham

Kate Pierson

Katherine Kelly Lang

James Brolin

Joe Montana

Joe Profit

John D. Rockefeller

John Robbins

John Stockton

Johnnetta Cole

"Most injuries require chiropractic care. It works better for me than anything else."

Jerry Rice

Johnny Damon

Joseph Arvay

Keith Crawford

Ken Berry

Kenny Sousa

Kim Basinger

Kim Kardashian

Lance Armstrong

Lenny McGill

Linda Hamilton

Lou Greenwood

Lucille Ball

Lynn Adams

Lynn Connelly

Mac Wilkins

Macaulay Culkin

Madonna

Mahatma Gandhi

Marcello Angelini

Marlo Thomas

Mark McGwire

Mark Portugal

Martina Navratilova

Mary Lou Retton

Mel Gibson

Mike Ingram

Jose Canseco

Josephine Premice-Fales

Keith Jackson

Kenny Loggins

Kevin Levrone

Kim Bauer (pro tennis player)

Kirt Manwaring

Lee Haney

Lester Archambeau

Liza Minnelli

Lou Waters

Members of Bon Jovi

Michael Jordan

Members of Extreme

Members of Grateful Dead

Mary Jo Peppler

Meredith Baxter

Michael Carbajal

Michael Jordan

Mark May

Maria Maricich (Olympic skier)

Mark Victor Hansen

Mary Decker

Matt LeBlanc

Michael Shurtleff

Mike Timson

"Chiropractic has advanced tremendously over the past few decades. It has become a specialized and accepted science."

Andy Griffith

Mindy Mylrea
Montel Williams
Nancy Ditz
Patrick Stewart
Patti Rizzo
Paul Frase
Penny Marshall
Peter Frampton
Richard Gere
Richard Pryor
Rick Valente
Robby Thompson
Robert Parish
Robin Williams
Rocky Marciano
Rosanne Cash
Ruffin Hamilton
Sally Little
San Francisco 49ers team
Scottie Pippen
Shaq
Sid Crosby
Suzy Chaffee
Tea Leoni

Monta Ellis
Muhammad Ali
Olga Korbut
Patrick Swayze
Patty Sheehan
Paul McCartney
Peter Fonda
Phyllis Diller
Richard Kuss
Rick Monday
Ricky Bell
Robert Goulet
Roberta Flack
Robin Wright
Roger Craig
Rudy Vallee
Ryan Sandberg
San Francisco Ballet
Sandra Palmer
Sean Landeta
Shirley MacLaine
Steven Seagal
Sylvester Stallone
Ted Danson

"Emmitt Smith Attributes His Success to Chiropractic"

Dallas Morning News, October 26, 2002

Terance Mathis
Terry Kirby
The Beach Boys
The Eagles
Tiger Woods
Tim Dwight
Tina Turner
Tom Brady
Tony Lopez
Toronto Maple Leafs team
Toronto Raptors team
Travis Tritt

Van Halen
Venus Williams
Victoria Williams
Wade Boggs Band
Warren Moon
Wayne Gretzky
Wes Parker
Whitney Houston
Whoopi Goldberg
William Holden
Willie Banks
Zach Johnson

"I have been going to chiropractors for as long as I can remember. It is as important to my training as the practice of my swing."

Tiger Woods

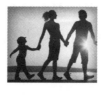

APPENDIX B

Patient Testimonials

Note: Check out the dozens of testimonies on video, organized by condition, on our website at UpperCervicalCare.com.

ADHD

Robin, Dillon's mom

When Dillon was three, he was evaluated and found to be "developmentally delayed" and diagnosed with ADHD (Attention Deficit Hyperactivity Disorder). He was placed in a special class, and his behavior was so difficult, uncontrollable really, that I had decided to ask his pediatrician about medication for his ADHD. Although I knew the side effects could be profound, I was exhausted and at my wits' end. My mother suggested I take Dillon to see Dr. Paul, an Upper Cervical Chiropractor, which I did. After Dillon's first Upper Cervical adjustment, he slept soundly through the night for the first time in his life. Each adjustment brought more milestones. Dillon began giving me hugs and kisses. By the beginning of the next school year, Dillon was a happy, healthy four-year-old and a joy to be around. His teachers were stunned. Now Dillon meets all his goals at school in record time. Dillon's life will never be the same, thanks to Upper Cervical.

Allergies/Hay Fever

David Mayer

Growing up, I had just about every kind of allergy you can think of. I was even allergic to the needles the doctors used to give me allergy shots. When I went to the draft board, because I was wheezing, they asked me, "Are you always like this?" I said, "No, this is my best day this year." They said, "We don't want you. We want to win the war." So, I went back to college and started working part-time for a chiropractor who gave me an atlas adjustment. I didn't know anything about chiropractors, but after two months, my hay fever and allergies completely went away. I changed my major from pre-dental to chiropractic. That was over 50 years ago. I was sick for 21 years, but I haven't been sick in the last 29.

Arthritis

Pat D.

When I was in my early fifties I noticed my arm and shoulder felt sore to the touch. It wasn't a throbbing pain, but if I rolled over on it while sleeping, it would wake me up. Then I had trouble opening jars. A few months later, I couldn't zip my dress in the back. I had to support one hand with the other to even lift a pan. Finally, I went to the doctor. Diagnosis: rheumatoid arthritis. He prescribed Celebrex and told me a lot of people my age "got arthritis." I didn't want to accept that. I was already going to an Upper Cervical doctor, but not regularly. Until the arthritis, I didn't think I needed to because I felt good most of the time. But I decided to stop taking the Celebrex and get back under regular Upper Cervical Care. Within six months, the arthritis was gone. I knew it was gone when the soreness left and I could, once again, do the yoga postures I'd done for years. I'm 65 now and still no arthritis. I do, however, go to Dr. Drury for regular upper cervical checkups. I learned that just because you feel good doesn't mean you're in alignment. An ounce of prevention is worth a pound of cure.

Back Pain

Dean M.

I've had low back pain all my life. I've worked over 20 years as a postal worker, standing on my feet for eight-plus hours a day. A friend referred me to Dr. Baker, an Upper Cervical chiropractor, for my pain. When Dr. Baker started X-raying my neck, I reminded him that it was my back that hurt, not my neck. He just smiled and explained again how Upper Cervical works. I felt immediate relief after my very first adjustment, and I was able to walk out of Dr. Baker's office better than I came in. After four weeks of Upper Cervical Care, I didn't have any back pain at all and haven't had any since. It's been over a year now, and I go see Dr. Baker once a month to make sure my adjustments are holding. My wife and my grandchildren and I are grateful for Upper Cervical Care and Dr. Baker.

Bed Wetting

Mother in KY

Our 15-year-old son was so embarrassed about his nightly incontinence that he would cry and beg to skip school. He retreated from everyone. Following his Upper Cervical correction, the incontinence diminished, and over a few weeks disappeared completely!

Bell's Palsy

Melissa

When I first came to Upper Cervical Health Centers, I came explicitly [because of] Bell's Palsy. I listed all the things that were wrong with me, and we got started. For seven years, I would have bowel movements maybe once a month. Ten minutes after my first Upper Cervical adjustment, I had a bowel movement. The Bell's Palsy was completely better within four weeks. Thank you, Upper Cervical.

Carpal Tunnel Syndrome

Patricia D.

I'd worn wrist braces for carpal tunnel; I'd even had carpal tunnel surgery, but nothing helped. I heard about Upper Cervical and said, "Why not?" although I have to admit I had my doubts about going to a chiropractor. At the time I'm giving this testimonial, I've been coming to

Upper Cervical Health Centers for five weeks and have had two adjustments. I don't know how to explain it, but I feel so much better. I feel my body is coming around and getting healthier.

Crossed Eyes (Strabismus)

Maria

In 1991, I was driving my car when I got rear-ended. Because I am short, the seat belt pulled tightly across my neck. The following year I noticed in a photo that the pupil of my left eye was off-center. After a time, my vision started being affected. Over the next 11 years I went to nine different doctors. My husband and I spent over $40,000 out of pocket on my medical treatments, and we had health insurance. We felt like we were just working for the doctors. I was prescribed different medications, but nothing helped. I had pain, too, but the pain was easier to deal with than my crossed eye. I felt very self-conscious. I wore a patch for a long time, because without it, both my vision and my balance were off. I even left one job to take another within walking distance of my home; I didn't trust my vision to drive. When a friend recommended Upper Cervical, I thought, well, all I have to lose is more money, so why not? I started seeing Dr. Drury in 2003. The first thing that happened was the pain went away—the feeling that someone was pulling my head back, the neck and shoulder pain—it all went away. About three-four months later, my eye was no longer crossed. Now I know when I need an adjustment; I get pain in my neck. I know if I don't get adjusted, my *eye will cross again. After Dr. Drury adjusts me, the pain goes away, and my eyes get stronger. Dr. Drury believes the injury from the seatbelt caused the trauma to my eye, and I do, too, although none of the medical doctors thought there was a connection between my accident and my eye. All I know is Upper Cervical helped me when nothing else could. I tell people to try Upper Cervical Care. Maybe it will help them, too.*

Degenerative Disc

Teri

Before I became an Upper Cervical patient of Dr. Weaver's in 2006, it was not unusual for me to miss work, a week at a time, because of back pain. I had been to all kinds of medical doctors, general chiropractors, neurologists, orthopedic surgeons, osteopaths, and acupuncturists, but I just kept getting worse. My first Upper Cervical adjustment brought immediate relief from the pain I walked in with that day, and after about six months under Upper Cervical Care, I missed only an occasional day of work because of back pain. I believe if I had not gotten under Upper Cervical Care that I would be totally disabled today. Now I'm functional. I'm working full-time, and I'm enjoying my life. I consider Upper Cervical Care to be the central part of my physical care, and I will be forever grateful.

Depression

Allie

When I first came to Dr. Hall, I was at the end of my rope. I was having terrible depression and anxiety, insomnia, and sometimes tingling and numbness in my hands and feet. I went to probably a half-dozen specialists all over the United States from Washington to Cedars-Sinai, but nobody was able to help me. I was diagnosed with everything from clinical depression to multiple sclerosis. Dr. Hall examined my neck and showed me how my atlas was twisted. When I was a very young boy, I fell off a donkey onto my neck. Dr. Hall did a correction, and I'd say after 10 to 15 minutes, it felt like somebody poured menthol all through my nerves, and I started to relax for the first time in probably 20 years. I've started to live again. The pain, the anxiety, the depression has completely gone away, and the sleeping is so much better. I can't recommend Upper Cervical Care enough. It saved my life, and I mean that literally.

Phil

When I came to see Dr. Drury for Upper Cervical Care, I'd been going to psychiatrists for four or five years. I never really got a diagnosis; they just give you medication after medication. At one time, I was on eight different pills. One prescription cost $30 a pill. They never said stop taking that one and start taking this one; they just kept adding new ones. I was in a really deep depression. I didn't want to do anything, had no interest in anything. After about *a month of Upper Cervical Care, I could tell my depression was lifting. Other people noticed, too, told me I was smiling more. I could tell I was feeling happier inside. The change was more gradual for me than it was Marge, my wife. Her neck pain went away the first time Dr. Drury adjusted her. We've been under Upper Cervical Care for over 10 years now, and we drive almost an hour to get here. People ask us why we don't go to a chiropractor in the town where we live. I tell them, "Because they're not Upper Cervical." Upper Cervical works.*

Ear Infection

Laura, Matthew's mom

Upper Cervical had helped me when I injured my back at work, but I never dreamed it would play such a crucial role in the healing of our young son. When Matthew was 10 days old, I noticed a "rattle" in his nose, which his pediatrician diagnosed as congestion. It turned into a sinus infection for which the doctor prescribed antibiotics. That led to a year and a half of constantly going to doctor visits because of bad ear infections. Matthew wasn't in day care or around cigarette smoke, and he was breast fed—the things that were supposed to prevent respiratory and ear problems. The pediatrician continued to prescribe antibiotics, and eventually Matthew was on breathing treatments around the clock, which led to surgery, having tubes put in his ears. During another round of testing, the pediatrician discovered Matthew's white blood cell count was exceptionally high and his red cell count low. By this time, Matthew had been on 19 rounds of antibiotics. During one of my Upper Cervical appointments, I was surprised to read in the literature that chiropractic can help ear infections, so I took Matthew to see Dr. Rob. Matthew was 14 months old when he received his first Upper Cervical adjustment. Within hours, his nose started to drain. I cried with joy. When Matthew's pediatrician tested his blood the following Tuesday, he said, "It's a miracle! Matthew's blood cell counts are normal!" I knew it wasn't a miracle. It was Upper Cervical. Matthew was completely healed in a few months. He's five now and is not bothered by sinus or ear problems, and he's never had another antibiotic, thanks to Upper Cervical Care.

Endometriosis

Mandy F.

I'd suffered from endometriosis since I was 14. I'd tried many different medications, treatments, even surgery to find relief from this painful, debilitating condition. I had such success with Dr. Broome, my Upper Cervical doctor, that now our whole family is under Upper Cervical Care. My husband was in constant pain from his work as a heavy equipment operator. Now he and both our sons are under Upper Cervical Care and getting the same great results I got. Upper Cervical Health Care has saved my marriage and my family.

Fibromyalgia

Avelica

After Upper Cervical Care, I'm almost pain-free, and I'd been in almost constant pain the last 10 years. I've been to many chiropractors, and Upper Cervical Care definitely works differently. I've never gotten the kind of relief that I got from Upper Cervical. I got relief after the very first Upper Cervical correction, and that had never happened with other chiropractors. I'd recommend Upper Cervical to anybody looking for relief from pain.

Gastric Reflux

Laura W.

For 27 years I suffered from chronic gastric reflux. I took two pills in the morning and two at night. In addition, I was on thyroid medication for over 20 years and on anti-depressants for the last three. I was a full-fledged skeptic about chiropractic, but after just two Upper Cervical adjustments with Dr. DiGregorio the pain is gone. Now I am medicine-free. I take nothing but vitamins!

General Pain

Agnes B.

When I first came to Dr. Dunsworth, I was skeptical and desperate. I was in so much pain I could hardly walk; I couldn't hold on to objects, and I was having trouble sleeping. I was thinking major surgery might be my only hope of getting better. Not only that, I was a single mom, and I couldn't afford to waste any more money trying to get better. I'd been to physical therapists, general chiropractors, and an acupuncturist. I was ready to start looking into applying for disability, the pain was so debilitating. But Upper Cervical has given me a second chance at life. What I got back was well worth the cost. Now my son is under Upper Cervical Care, too. He hasn't been sick since he had his first Upper Cervical adjustment seven months ago. I am so grateful to Dr. Dunsworth. Now that I don't have to deal with pain every day, I can be the mom I wasn't able to be before Upper Cervical.

Headaches/Migraines

Alatha C.

I had severe headaches for 15 years and sought help from my family physician who sent me to a neurologist. All the doctors gave me medication with side effects that made me feel even worse. After my first Upper Cervical adjustment, I saw amazing results. Headaches are now rare, and I have more energy to enjoy life. X-rays on my first Upper Cervical visit showed the problem, and healing started. Thank you, Dr. Christine Theodossis!

Alyssa

I had headaches every single day of my life. After one Upper Cervical correction, my headaches went away. I sing, so I went for a voice lesson the day I got adjusted, and we started doing exercises. My voice teacher was amazed, because I'd gained an octave in my voice! She couldn't believe it. Now my voice teacher wants to see my Upper Cervical doctor. My whole family, my parents and grandparents, are now under Upper Cervical Care. I give out Dr. Wagner's card to everybody I can.

Mandy F.

I've had migraine headaches since I was a teenager. I've treated them with antidepressants, antihypertensives, antiseizure medications, steroid infusions, lumbar punctures, numerous CT scans, and MRIs. Every treatment ended in disappointment. A friend recommended Dr. Broome, an Upper Cervical doctor. At the time, I was living in survival mode, so I figured I didn't have much to lose. That was two and a half years ago, I had no idea how Upper Cervical would change my life. I will be forever grateful to Dr. Broome and Upper Cervical Care.

Herniated Disc

Carl

I woke up one morning and could hardly move. I went to my medical doctor who told me I had a herniated disc. He said I needed an operation and wanted to schedule it right away. My wife said, "Okay, let's schedule it, but let's also go see another doctor for a second opinion." The second doctor told me I didn't need an operation, but I'd have to have a shot that would bring relief for two to three weeks. Then I'd get another shot. That didn't seem like a good idea, so I went to a third doctor. He told me I needed to do these exercises, but I could hardly move, much less exercise. My wife's hairdresser told her about this Upper Cervical doctor who'd helped her, so I went to him. After one month of care with Dr. Hall, not only did the herniated disc go away; I used to have chronic pain across my back and that disappeared, too. I didn't need an operation. I can bend, walk, even garden without pain. Now I'm coming to Dr. Hall to try to reduce my blood pressure, which has come down. I want to get off my blood pressure medicine.

Hip and Knee Pain

Barbara

I'm in my sixties and was having a lot of pain in my hip and knee when I came to Upper Cervical Health Centers. When I first came in, I was a little afraid they might hurt my neck, but they didn't. After being under Upper Cervical just a month, my knee pain is completely gone and my hip pain is getting better. Not only that, when I came in, I was sleeping maybe two hours a night. Now I'm sleeping five hours before waking up, which is amazing to me. Upper Cervical has helped me so much. I just want other people to know about it, so they can benefit. I know a lot of people have knee problems like I did.

Infertility

Annette

I started having trouble with my menstrual cycle at age 12. My mother took me to medical doctors, but they couldn't find anything wrong with me. When I got married, we eventually adopted a beautiful little boy as it seemed we weren't going to have our own children. I'd been married 15 years when I got under Upper Cervical Care with Dr. Holliday. Three months later, I was pregnant. I had a son. The month he turned one, I found out I was pregnant again! Upper Cervical fixed a problem medical doctors could not, and I have three beautiful sons to prove it.

Injury from Fall

Gina Y.

Our eight-year-old son, Kyle, fell sideways off a ladder. His head hit the concrete with a sickening thud. We immediately called 911, and Kyle was rushed to the hospital. An MRI showed that Kyle had a skull fracture. He had a pocket of fluid on the side of his head that was leaking out through the fracture in his skull. Kyle was in a lot of pain and couldn't walk or sit up. After four days in the hospital, we took Kyle home. The doctors told us it would take two, three months for Kyle to recover. After 10 days of Kyle lying flat on his back with no improvement, I decided to take him to see Dr. Schurger, my Upper Cervical doctor. I had gotten amazing results with Upper Cervical and felt confident that Dr. Schurger's specialized adjustment would help Kyle's body heal faster. After the diagnostic X-rays, Dr. Schurger adjusted the top two bones in Kyle's neck that were severely misaligned. Kyle felt no pain and slept soundly for 30 minutes after the adjustment. Much to my amazement, Kyle left Dr. Schurger's office walking on his own! When we got home, Kyle started running and playing like nothing had happened. He didn't take any pain medication after that day, and all the swelling was gone 24 hours after his Upper Cervical correction. We are so grateful to God for leading us to Dr. Schurger.

Insomnia

Heather

My daughter suffered from insomnia. It would take her hours to fall asleep only to wake up during the night. She would cry and become very upset because she was so tired all the time. After her first Upper Cervical adjustment with Dr. DiGregorio, she slept through the night. She was able to fall asleep shortly after going to bed and never woke up during the night. She continues to sleep through the night.

Irritable Bowel Syndrome

Patty

People who have irritable bowel syndrome don't talk about it much, because, well, it's embarrassing. Who wants to tell people that they can't go out to dinner or they weren't at the birthday party because they were afraid when they ate, their stomach would start cramping and they'd have to make a beeline for the bathroom? My life has been pretty much controlled by IBS since I was a child. I couldn't control my bowels, so I just tried to cope by staying home in a safe environment and eating very little. Living with IBS is horrific.

When a friend recommended Upper Cervical, I didn't really believe in chiropractors. But he assured me the adjustment wouldn't hurt, so I went. I remember eating after my first Upper Cervical adjustment and not getting sick. I thought, "Holy Moly, that's amazing!" That was about three and a half years ago. Now my corrections are holding a month or longer, and I go six months at a time without an IBS episode. That has been life-changing for me. It's wonderful to be able to be around people and not have to worry. I went back to my gastro doctor and told him he should tell his patients about Upper Cervical Care.

Ménière's Disease

Peter L.

I started experiencing vertigo and couldn't function in my work as a pilot. I went to a medical doctor; general chiropractor; and an ear, nose, and throat specialist. Nothing helped. A friend told us about Upper Cervical, and I found an Upper Cervical doctor about 30 minutes from where we lived. After my second Upper Cervical adjustment, I got my balance back, no vertigo. It was totally amazing. After about a month, I started flying again. It was a miracle to be able to go back to what I was doing.

Multiple Sclerosis

Karen B.

About four years ago, I hurt my neck really bad in a car accident. They told me I had whiplash and that it would go away in a couple of weeks. Two years later, I started getting shooting pains down my left arm and leg with muscle weakness. The doctors told me I had multiple sclerosis! I was only 22 years old. Furthermore, they told me there was no cure, but they could give me medicine to help with the pain until I died. Over the next two years, I kept getting worse. I could barely move my left leg. I couldn't drive, and I could no longer work. I had difficulty sleeping. My cousin told me to go see Dr. Baker, an Upper Cervical doctor, which I did. Within eight weeks, I was back to normal and all my symptoms were gone. Now, I work, I go dancing, I work out! Thank you, Dr. Baker, for giving me my life back.

Neck Pain

Joe

I was working with another chiropractor with a different philosophy. I liked the guy, and I was making some progress, but the pain came back a couple of days after my adjustments. I was on my way to Mayo Clinic because the pain had got so intense when I was referred to Dr. Hunt, an Upper Cervical chiropractor. I felt relief after my first adjustment. After my sixth Upper Cervical correction, I'd say my pain went from a level 10 to a level two or three. About my tenth visit, I was having zero pain. I can't tell you how much better I feel.

Donnie

I'm 70 years old. I woke up one morning and thought I had a crick in my neck, but it didn't go away. For two, three months, I couldn't turn my neck. My medical doctor

*X-rayed it and told me I had a pinched nerve. He sent
me home with a bunch of drugs, but I still couldn't turn
my neck. Then I went to Upper Cervical Health Centers,
and after six Upper Cervical visits, I could turn my neck,
which means I can drive again, because I can turn my
neck to look over my shoulder.*

Anne

*When I met Dr. Knecht at the Edwardsville Farmer's
Market, I asked him, with only a glimmer of hope, if
Upper Cervical would help my neck pain. At the time,
I had a hard time doing simple things like running the
vacuum and pushing a grocery cart. I'd tried just about
everything including physical therapy, over-the-counter
pain relievers, homeopathic and herbal medicine, but
nothing seemed to help. Two days after my first Upper
Cervical adjustment, I was gardening! I haven't had
to take anything for pain for over eight months now. I
couldn't believe that Upper Cervical worked, and especially, I couldn't believe that it lasted. Our whole family—my husband and I and our nine children, ages six
to 26—is now under Upper Cervical Care. The change
has been so wonderful and dramatic. What if I'd never
discovered Upper Cervical Care?*

Pain from Old Injuries

Sean

*I've suffered from pain for over 20 years. I spent most of
my life in the military and was an ejection seat trainer in*

the Navy. I've been in a lot of search-and-rescue missions and suffered from all kinds of fractures. My body has been injured a lot over time. I was relying on heavy-duty narcotics like oxycotin to deal with the pain, which was 24/7. I had taken so many over-the-counter painkillers that I developed an ulcer. When I saw Upper Cervical on the Internet, I thought it sounded different. It made sense to me, so I decided to try it. Since I've been coming to Dr. Drury for Upper Cervical Care, I've had more days without pain than with pain, and that's amazing for me. My insomnia is getting better; my gastro-intestinal problems are getting better. I'm very pleased and looking forward to continuing Upper Cervical Care.

Peripheral Neuropathy

Deborah

I had tingling and numbness in my hands and feet and was in a lot of pain. I found out about Upper Cervical Care at a home show in Illinois. After Upper Cervical adjustments, the pain and numbness miraculously went away. I knew I was healing the day I was able to pick up a 12-inch, cast iron skillet with one hand. I had strength I hadn't had before. I can do so much more now than I used to be able to do. I'd recommend anybody and everybody to get checked by an Upper Cervical doctor, because it's simply amazing, the results.

Sciatica

Pilar R.
(An Italian American who sought Upper Cervical help
while in Rome)

I had a motorcycle accident when I was 13, which I think caused my severe sciatica many years later. I'd tried chiropractic care, cortisone shots, and acupuncture. When those things didn't help I had surgery on my lower back at Lenox Hill Hospital in NYC. I felt better for a while, but my entire posture was changed for the worse, and nine months later, I was in pain again, and I walked with a severe limp. I have to use a cane. Doctors didn't know what was wrong with me. With one month of Upper Cervical Care, I can walk straight with no limp. I take long walks again, and my posture has significantly improved. After each adjustment, I feel renewed with a sense of well-being that I've not felt for a long time. I am honestly surprised by the results I get from this technique. I'm happy to have discovered Upper Cervical Care with Dr. Cormier and will continue to be an Upper Cervical patient when I get back to the states.

Scoliosis

Meryl

I was diagnosed with scoliosis at age 11. I couldn't do a lot of things like other kids. I'd go to doctors and they'd give me muscle relaxers. I also had a damaged nerve in my arm, which doctors told me would eventually require surgery. It hurt to use my arm. After I started going to

Dr. Wagner for Upper Cervical Care, my scoliosis got better, the pain in my arm went away, and allergies that I'd always been bothered with disappeared. Now, when my allergies start acting up, I know I'm out of alignment and it's time to go see Dr. Wagner. Upper Cervical works.

Sinus

Jessica

For 15 years, I had sinus issues. I had daily headaches and I was congested all the time. My mother made my appointment with Dr. Monnin for Upper Cervical Care. I went reluctantly thinking there's no way this is going to help. About six hours after my first correction, my headache was gone, and I actually had a runny nose— something unheard of for me. At my next appointment, I admitted to Dr. Monnin that I'd been skeptical. After my correction, while lying in the resting room, my ears started popping and within a few hours, I felt amazing. Now I can tell Dr. Monnin if I'm going to need a correction before he scans; my symptoms are that exact. My ear, nose, and throat doctor used to talk to me about having sinus surgery. I'm so glad I decided against it. I'd recommend Upper Cervical to anyone. I just wish I'd found it sooner.

TMJ

Ruth

One day I woke up with pain on one side of my face. Then I started having pain and numbness on my forehead and pain in my neck and the back of my head. I would go to the emergency room, but nobody knew what it was. I went to all kinds of doctors and specialists. Finally, one of them told me TMJ was causing my symptoms. I was in pain all the time. I have four kids, and I wasn't able to play with them; I couldn't even read to them. My husband watched them as much as he could, so I could sleep. It was a very stressful time in my life, in all our lives. I had a feeling like I was under water and couldn't get air. I know that sounds crazy, but I felt like I had no oxygen in my head. The very first time Dr. Hall gave me an Upper Cervical adjustment, it felt like all this air rushed back into my head. My eyes were brighter. It took awhile. I came to Dr. Hall twice a week for a month, then once a week. Slowly, the pain started going away, one area at a time. I'd say after six months or so, all the pain was gone, 100% gone, and it hasn't come back. I come see Dr. Hall now for maintenance. I used to cry every time I came in to see Dr. Hall. I haven't done that in a long time. Upper Cervical gave me my life back.

Tourette's

Parent

My son Dayton developed Tourette syndrome a couple of months after being hit in the head by a foul softball. The doctors told us the tics may have started because of the concussion from the hit, but there was nothing they could do. We chose not to medicate, but a few years later, I contemplated reconsidering when the tics started get-ting worse. Then one day, I stumbled upon a website of an Upper Cervical chiropractor. On the website, there were stories of other children with Tourette syndrome and how they'd gotten better under Upper Cervical Care. After Dr. Muths gave Dayton his first Upper Cervical adjustment, I noticed about a 95% decrease in his tics, and since then, Dayton's gone several weeks without tics. Dayton continues to get Upper Cervical corrections. This has been a miracle to him. It has changed his life.

Tinnitus

Pat A.

I had tinnitus so bad I thought I was going to have to retire, and I wasn't ready to retire. I was losing my balance and getting deafer by the minute. Now, I'm a psychotherapist and I'm also a doubter. I guess I want people to know that I'm an intelligent person with access to quality information. If I hadn't experienced it, I wouldn't have thought Upper Cervical adjustments could make that kind of difference in my health. After three months under Upper Cervical Care, I have no symptoms of tinnitus, and I feel more stable than I can remember feeling in my life.

Transverse Myelitis

Danny R.

In August of 2007, I was diagnosed with an autoimmune disease called Transverse Myelitis. I had numbness in my feet and legs along with a severe burning sensation in my heels. My primary physician sent me to a neurologist who did multiple tests including three MRIs. I was prescribed gabapentin, tramadol, and Vioxx. These drugs really reduced my pain. I thought I was in heaven until the side effects kicked in. Then I became a different person: dull, tired, slow, and cloudy. My neurologist also suggested a steroid IV injection, and a nurse came to my house to administer the IV. The results seemed miraculous. I played golf for the first time in months. However, another wave of side effects followed that I could never have prepared for. I had unprovoked anger, emotional breakdowns, and intense frustration, which led to isolation. It was easier to stay home than to deal with people.

One day a friend came to my house to sit with me while I was "hooked up." He brought me several books to read, and one of them was James Tomasi's What Time Tuesday? *I read the book, and although I was still skeptical about this miraculous Upper Cervical Care Tomasi wrote about, I decided to call Upper Cervical Health Centers of America to find an Upper Cervical doctor near me. The first time the Upper Cervical doctor adjusted me, I felt nothing, which heightened my skepticism. However, I knew I couldn't stay on these drugs forever, so I stuck with Upper Cervical. Well, I eventually got off all the drugs while experiencing, what I would estimate, a 95% reduction in my pain. I am thankful for the job Upper Cervical doctors do and will forever be indebted to their dedication and ability to help my body heal itself.*

Trigeminal Neuralgia

Susan K.

The pain I suffered from TN was so traumatic I hesitate to talk about it. It was unrelenting for 15 years. I took so much ibuprofen that I burned out the lining of my intestinal system.

I underwent surgery at Mayo Clinic in 2008. While I was in intensive care, the surgeon told me he had found nothing wrong with me. I went home with 22 staples in the back of my head and increased pain. I found Upper Cervical from a Google Search for "cures for trigeminal neuralgia." It was with extreme skepticism that I went to see Dr. Troyer, an Upper Cervical doctor near me. After a few Upper Cervical corrections, I was off all neurological medications plus the Nexium I was taking for my stomach. I don't hurt anymore. I enjoy life now, something I haven't done for 15 years.

* For more testimonials or more information on Upper Cervical Care, or to find an Upper Cervical doctor near you, please visit our website at www.BestKeptSecretInHealthCare.com.

WORKS CITED

1 World Health Report. *Photius.* 2000. web. 3 August
    2012.

2 Smith, Kathryn. *Politico.* n.p., 3 May 2012. web. 3
    August 2012.

3 Wilk, Chester. *Medicine, Monopolies, and Malice.*
    Chicago: n.p. 1996. Print.

4 Zennie, Michael. *Dailymail.com.* 10 May 2012. web.
    26 Nov. 2012.

5 Kent, Christoher. *Mercola.com.* 15 Jan. 2008. web.
    24 Oct. 2012.

6 *Your Health.* "Injury Prevention." 3 March 2011.
    web. 24 October 2012.

7 Thompson, Dennis. *HealthDay. US News and World
    Report.* 29 Dec. 2009. web. 24 Oct. 2012.

8 Johnson, Linda A. *USA Today.* 4 April 2012. web. 3
    August 2012.

9 Peterson, Melody. *Our Daily Meds.* New York:
    Farrar, Strauss and Giroux, 2009. Print.

10 Ibid.

11 Makary, Marty, MD. "How to Stop Hospitals from
    Killing Us." *The Wall Street Journal.* 22 Sept.
    2012. web. 14 November 2012.

12 Weinberger, Jill. *CNBC.com.* 23 May 2011. web. 26
    Nov. 2012.

13 Goldhill, David. *Catastrophic Care.* New York;
    Alfred A. Knopf. 2013. Print.

14 Ibid.

15 Reed, Deoine, PhD. and Kemmerly, Sandra, MD. "Infection Control and Prevention: A Review of Hospital-Acquired Infections and the Economic Implications." *The Ochsner Journal*. 9(Spring 2009) 27-31. web.

16 *Alliance for Human Research Protection*. "U.S. Health Care Third Leading Cause of Death." 15 Sept. 2000. web. 24 Oct. 2012.

17 Szabo, Liz. *USA Today*. 30 July 2009. web. 3 July 2012.

18 Eriksen, Kirk. *Upper Cervical Subluxation Complex—A Complete Review of Chiropractic and Medical Literature*. Philadelphia: Lippincott, Williams, and Wilkins, 2004. Print.

19 *The Spinal Column*. Upper Cervical Health Centers' Newsletter, March 2012.

20 Quigley, W.H. "Pioneering Mental Health: Institutional Psychiatric Care." *Chiropractic History*. 3. (1983): 69-75. web. 27 Nov. 12.

21 Frigard, L. Ted. "Dr. Palmer vs. Dr. Mayo." *Dynamic Chiropractic*. 12 June 2000. web. 27 August 2012.

22 Chiroeco, David D. Palmer: *Chiropractic's Educator*. web. 20 August 2012.

23 Rand Objective Analysis. Effective Solutions. *Changing Views of Chiropractic and a National Reappraisal of Nontraditional Health Care Research Brief*. web. 16 September 2010.

24 Dye, A.A. *The Evolution of Chiropractic—Its Discovery and Development*. Richmond Hill, NY: Richmond Hall, 1939. Print.

25 Keating, Joseph, PhD. "The Meaning of Innate." *Journal of Canadian Chiropractic Association.* 46 (March 2002); 4-9. Print.

26 *We Create Wellness.* Optimal Wellness Center. 26 Feb. 2009. web. 27 Aug. 2012.

27 Palmer, B. J. *The Subluxation Specific— The Adjustment Specific.* Davenport, Iowa: The Palmer School of Chiropractic, 1934. Print.

28 Eriksen, Kirk. *Upper Cervical Subluxation Complex—A Complete Review of Chiropractic and Medical Literature.* Philadelphia: Lippincott, Williams, and Wilkins, 2004. Print.

29 Smith, R. "Where Is the Wisdom?" *British Medical Journal.* 303. (1991): 798-799. Print.

30 Ioannidis, John. "Why Most Published Research Findings Are False." *Chance.* 18 (2005) 4. web. 29 Nov, 2012.

31 Angell, Marcia, MD. *The Truth about Drug Companies: How They Deceive Us and What to Do About It.* New York: Random House, 2004.

32 *World Health Organization.* 2012. web. 22 August 2012.

33 The International Chiropractic Pediatric Association. *ICPA4kids.com.* "Chiropractic Care for Children Is Safe and Effective." ICPA, 17 Sept. 2009. web. 11 Sept. 2012.

34 Reuters. *Rense.com.* 19 Sept. 2002. web. 12 Sept. 2012.

35 Health Day News. *MedlinePlus.* U.S. National Library of Medicine, National Institutes of Health. 18 June 2012. web. 12 Sept. 2012.

36 Wickens, Pearce, Crane, and Beasley. "Antibiotics Use in Early Childhood and the Development of Asthma." *Clinical Experimental Allergy*. 1999. 30(11): 1547-1553.

37 Eriksen, Kirk. *Upper Cervical Subluxation Complex – A Complete Review of Chiropractic and Medical Literature*. Philadelphia: Lippincott, Williams, and Wilkins, 2004. Print.

38 Vallone, Sharon. "Linking Craniocervical Subluxation in Infants with Breastfeeding Difficulties." *International Chiropractic Association*. 53. (1997): 42-48. Print.

39 Klougart, Nilsson and Jacobsen. "Infantile Colic Treated by Chiropractors: A Prospective Study of 316 Cases." *Journal of Manipulative Physiological Therapy*. 12. (1989): 281-288. Print.

40 Wilberg, Nordsteen, and Nilsson. "The Short-Term Effect of Spinal Manipulation in the Treatment of Infantile Colic." *Journal of Manipulative Physiological Therapy*. 22. (1999): 51-521. Print.

41 Donovan, Deb, and Vanmetter, Bob. "Is There a Brain Stem-SIDS Connection?" *ivillage*. 1 January, 1999. web. 3 Dec. 2012.

42 Eriksen, p. 55.

43 Ibid., p. 56.

44 Hendley, J.O. "Clinical Practice, Otitis Media." *New England Journal of Medicine*. 347 (2002): 1169-1174. Print.

45 Ericksen, p. 323.

46 "New Data on Autism Spectrum Disorders." *Centers

for Disease Control. 29 May 2012. web. 3 Dec. 2012.

47 Eriksen, p. 323.

48 Ibid., p. 292.

49 <u>Ibid</u>., p. 293.

50 Ressel, Ogi. "Health—Ritalin." *Alive.* web. 3 December 2012.

51 "Ritalin—Physicians' Desk Reference." *PDR Health.* 2011. web. 3 Dec. 2012.

52 Eriksen, p. 393.

53 Ibid., p. 386.

54 Ibid.

55 "Increasing Number of Children Receive Chiropractic Care." *American Chiropractic Association.* (Jan. 2009), web. 3 Dec. 2012.

56 Crossman, Ashley. *Sociology.About.com; The New York Times.* "The Social Traqnsformation of American Medicine." N.d. web. 28 August 2012.

57 Frigard, L. Ted. "Dr. Palmer vs. Dr. Mayo." *Dynamic Chiropractic.* 12 June 2000. web. 27 August 2012.

58 Wilk, Chester. *Medicine, Monopolies, and Malice.* Chicago, 1996. Print.

59 Ibid., pp. 67-68.

60 Ibid., p. 158.

61 Ibid., p. 126.

62 Susan Getzendanner, District Judge. *Wilk v. AMA.* 27 August 1987. "Statement of the American Chiropractic Association on the AMA Scope of Practice Partnership." *Acatoday.com./pdf/ACA-AMA. 1990. web.* 11 June 2012.

63 "High Court Favors P&G over Amway." *The Houston Chronicle.* 2 October 2001. web. 26 June 2012.

64 Wilk, Chester. *Medicine, Monopolies, and Malice.* Chicago, 1996. Print.

65 Harrison, Hugh. *The Man Who Made a Ladder of His Cross.* Davenport: n.p. 1919. Print.

66 Ibid.

67 Wilk, Chester. Dr. *Medicine, Monopolies, and Malice.* Chicago, 1996. Print.

68 Coulter, I., Adams, A., Coggan, P., Wilkesm M., Gonyea, M. "A Comparative Study of Chiropractic and Medical Education." *Alternative Medicine.* 4 (1998): 64-75. Print.

69 Freedman, KB, Bernstein, J. "The Adequacy of Medical School Education in Musculoskeletal Medicine." *Journal of Bone Joint Surgery.* 80-A. (1998): 1427. Print.

70 Eriksen, Kirk. *Upper Cervical Subluxation Complex – A Complete Review of Chiropractic and Medical Literature.* Philadelphia: Lippincott, Williams and Wilkins, 2004. Print.

71 Ibid., p. 416.

72 Ibid., p. 331.

73 Ibid., p. 345.

74 Stat, Terri Yablonsky. "Lower Blood Pressure with Neck Alignment." *The Chicago Tribune.* (8 May 2007): web.

75 DeNoon, Daniel. "Study Finds Atlas Adjustment Lowers Blood Pressure." *WebMD.* 16 March 2007. web. 19 September 2012.

76 Upton, AR and McComas, AJ. "The Double Crush in Nerve Entrapment Syndromes." *The Lancet.* 7825. (18 August 1973): 359-362. Print.

77 "Nervous System Appears to Play Key Role in Developing Type I Diabetes: Study." *Toronto Daily Press.* 15 December 2006. web. 4 December 2012.

78 Eriksen, p. 310.

79 Hoh, David. *Chronic Fatigue and Immune Dysfunction Syndrome Association of America.* May-June 1999. web. 4 December 2012.

80 "Fact Sheet." *National Headache Foundation.* web. 4 December 2012.

81 Eriksen, p. 262.

82 Ibid.

83 Ibid., p. 264.

84 Ibid., p. 267.

85 Ibid., p. 269.

86 Ibid., p. 276.

87 Ibid., p. 311.

88 Ibid., p. 314.

89 Poser, Charles. "Trauma to the Central Nervous System." *The JAMA Network, Archives of Neurology.* 57(7). July 2000. web. 4 December 2012.

90 Merceca, Guiseppe, MD and Mandolesi, Sandro, MD. Personal Interview. 5 May 2012.

91 Merceca, Guiseppe, MD and Mandolesi, Sandro. MD. "Preliminary Results Post Upper Cervical Treatment in Patients with Multiple Sclerosis and CCSVI." Upper Cervical Health

Centers' Annual Convention. Las Vegas. 5 May 2012.

92 Herzberg, Uri. "Chronic Pain and Immunity." *Science Direct.* 59 (2). Nov. 1994. web. 4 December 2012.

93 Eriksen, p. 98.

94 Ibid., p. 328.

95 Ibid., p.94.

96 Ibid., p. 280.

97 "Acute Low Back Problems in Adults."*Agency for Health Care Policy and Research.* No. 95-0642. (December 1994): p. 5. Print.

98 "Cost of Lumbar Surgery." *Spine-Health.* 25 July 2009. web. 3 October 2012.

99 "Famous Celebrities and Athletes under Chiropractic Care." *Chiro.cc.* web. 3 September 2012.